Praise for
Win the Weight War

Ten Successful Strategies for Taking It Off and Keeping It Off

As a business manager, I've noticed how often weight gain and problems on the job occur together. Resolving those job problems and returning to normal weight also seem to happen together. That's why I'm very happy with Jill's book. Follow Jill's strategies and your bathroom scale will measure both your weight and your self-leadership. Manage your weight, manage yourself. It's all in Jill's book.

John Buck, Certified Dynamic
Self-Governance Consultant,
"GovernanceAlive.com" Co-author of *We*
the People: Consenting to a Deeper Democracy.

I am a "baby-boomer" who is still struggling with a recent 10 pound weight gain following thyroid surgery. This book comes at a perfect time! I know my lifelong struggle against extra pounds will be even more challenging with age, and I need the kind of holistic approach which Jill Cody offers in her easy to read and understand book.

Sue Hecht, Maryland State
House of Delegates

"Win the Weight War" is not just another diet book with a structured food plan. Jill looks at all the angles that are roadblocks to long term success. You will be offered step-by step guidance on how to achieve life goals, unburdened by worries about your weight.

Heather Kaye, Life Coach, *Invision*

This is a book that explains how to fix the emotional blocks that stop you from winning that weight struggle. I loved it! Jill Cody explains it in ways that make sense and are easy to follow.

Susan Taylor President, S.
Taylor Collections

Winning the Weight Wars offers motivating, educational and practical strategies for winning the "battle of the bulge."

Judith E. Pearson, Ph.D. Clinical Counselor and Hypnotherapist, Author: *Weight, Hypnotherapy, and YOU*

Jill Cody has created an exciting and proven discipline to win your war on weight loss. If you are serious about succeeding in winning this personal battle, this book is a must read. You will finally emerge the victor in that elusive weight war you have been fighting!

Annelie Weber, Coach/Mentor

Win the Weight War is like a delicious tossed-salad starting with a base of principles of human behavior. Add main ingredients of personal stories, specific "how-to's, and realistic approaches to making life changes. Season with a conversational style as if Jill is talking just with you and top it all off with the A-B-C's of winning your personal weight war and resources for further study. Mix it all up in a bowl of positive approaches to "winning challenges" rather than "losing weight", and satisfy the craving for a unique approach to weight management.

Sylvia Henderson, Founder/ CEO - SpringboardTraining.com; Author; Speaker; Television Host

Wow! Jill's book is logical and easy to understand. I wish I had read this book ten years ago. It's a real recipe for success.

Audrey Komrad

It was so nice to read a book that finally put weight struggles into perspective. It is such a readable take on the problems so many people struggle to solve. The bottom line is those comfort foods just don't make it.

Martha White, Personal Trainer.

Win the Weight War

Win the Weight War

10 Transforming

Perspectives to **Take it off**

and **Keep it off**

Jill B. Cody, MA, L.C.P.C.

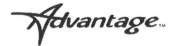

Published by Advantage, Charleston, South Carolina.
Member of Advantage Media Group.

ADVANTAGE is a registered trademark and the Advantage colophon is a trademark of Advantage Media Group, Inc.

Printed in the United States of America.

ISBN: 978-1-59932-051-9
LCCN: 2007906947

Most Advantage Media Group titles are available at special quantity discounts for bulk purchases for sales promotions, premiums, fundraising, and educational use. Special versions or book excerpts can also be created to fit specific needs.

For more information, please write: Special Markets, Advantage Media Group, P.O. Box 272, Charleston, SC 29402 or call 1.866.775.1696.

[The information contained in this book is not intended to serve as a replacement for professional medical advice. Any use of the information in this book is at the reader's discretion. The author and the publisher specifically disclaim any and all liability arising directly or indirectly from the use or application of any information contained in this book. A health care professional should be consulted regarding your specific situation or concerns.]

*Dedicated to the love of my life, my biggest fan, advocate, and personal cheerleader — my wonderful husband of forty-five years, **Richard Cody**. With his love and support, I can accomplish anything!*

Table of Contents

Foreword

Obesity has truly become an epidemic. According to the Centers for Disease Control and Prevention (CDC) 87.2 percent of all Americans is either overweight (60.5%), obese (23.9%) or grossly obese (3.0%). Wait read that again. 87.2 percent of us are—dare I say it—too fat! That's more than 90 percent of us! Or to put it in more positive terms, only about 1 in 10 of us weighs what we are supposed to weigh. (For details, go to http://www.cdc.gov/mmwr/preview/mmwrhtml/mm5536a1.htm.)

The bad news, despite a wide variety of healthcare initiatives, the prevalence of obesity, according to the CDC, continues to *increase* in *all* states. And the really bad news is that it costs all of us big time. First, it decreases the quality of our lives. For example, the CDC tells us that obesity is associated with increased risk for hypertension, dyslipidemia, type 2 diabetes, coronary heart disease, stroke and certain cancers. All nasty stuff that will not only shorten your life, but also will make you more miserable while you're still alive. But that's not all. It also costs us lots more in taxes. How much? According to one study reported by CDC, the state-specific obesity-attributable annual medical expenditures ranged from $87 million in Wyoming to—are you ready for this—$7.7 billion in California. Just think of how much better, longer and cheaper you and I could live if we got this obesity thing under control.

What to do? According to the CDC "the continued increase in obesity prevalence underscores the need for additional measures to educate and motivate persons to make healthier choices…" (http://www.cdc.gov/mmwr/preview/mmwrhtml/mm5536a1.htm)

The good news, that's exactly what this book will help you do! It will educate and motivate you to take actions that will enable *you* to take it off and keep it off!

But, you might say, I've read lots of diet books, and none of them have worked. I hear you. However, this book is different. Using an NLP framework, Jill Cody helps you address numerous emotional roadblocks that keep you stuck in your old thinking and eating habits. The main points in this book may seem obvious at first, but are extremely important in helping you be successful in winning the weight war. For example, one important message: *"Stop focusing on loss! Instead – look at what you want to* win," you'll want to put to work right now, because it will cause you to think and act more positive. And if you've read my powerful book *Make It a Winning Life—Success Strategies for Life, Love and Business*, then you already know that that one fail-safe transformation will empower you to take positive actions that will put you on the road to winning the weight war, right *now*.

In this easy-to-read book Jill, an experienced psychotherapist who has helped numerous clients successfully combat these overweight issues for over 25 years, teaches you 10 practical strategies to overcome old emotional "traps" that stand in your way of making consistent healthy choices.

The concept of creating an "internal ally," reinforced by specific examples of how other people have actually used Jill's strategies, will reinforce your enthusiasm and commitment to achieve your weight and/or size goal. You will be energized, motivated, and will truly appreciate the values and benefits of achieving the weight you want.

In short, this book will educate and motivate you to take actions to *take it off and keep it off* and *win the weight war* once and for all!

Wolf J. Rinke, PhD, RD, CSP

Author of several best selling books, audio and video programs including *Make It a Winning Life—Success Strategies for Life, Love and Business*

www.WolfRinke.com

Acknowledgements

There are many people I would like to acknowledge in the creation of this book. First and foremost, I want to thank **all my clients** who have shared their personal stories, and have been so enthusiastic about the progress they have made – and continue to make. You-all have been my biggest cheerleaders in my efforts to write this book. Indeed, this book is dedicated to all of you – past, present, and future.

A warm, heartfelt "thank you" goes to **Susan Taylor, Lorna House, Judy Pearson**, and **Audrey Komrad** for their help in reading the chapters, and making great suggestions. It really helped me get objective perspectives.

Ron Klein, the originator and prime mover of the **American Hypnosis Training Academy** has been my colleague, mentor, friend, and an NLP trainer par excellence. All his training, encouragement, critique and suggestions in my learning, and teaching NLP and Ericksonian Hypnosis as it relates to helping people control their weight have been invaluable.

A special thank you to my good friend, mentor and masterful web designer, **Georgia Patrick, "The Communicators"**, whose unwavering support, advice and encouragement has been priceless.

I want to especially recognize the contributions of **Benjamin Miller** who worked hard at editing and re-editing to make it right.

I especially want to express enthusiastic appreciation to my mentor, colleague and friend, **Wolf Rinke, PhD,** author of *Make It a Winning Life* for making substantive "winning" suggestions about the structure of the book, and for writing the Foreword.

I owe particular acknowledgement and appreciation to the contributions from my trainer, **Kip Jawish**, of **In-Fit Studios** whose energy and expertise helped to craft the chapter on physical fitness.

Jane Gross Mercado has been a wonderful friend and colleague since our years in graduate school, and our first ventures into the world of professional counseling. It is with great delight that I can appreciate all her wonderful help and suggestions in reading the manuscript, and getting as excited and enthused about the book as I was. Her chapter on healthy cooking strategies makes a wonderful addition to the book.

Introduction: Basic Winning Weight Strategies

Cookie! ... Cookie! ... That cookie is calling to me – and I must respond. If I don't get it, I will be a cranky, unpleasant person because I am *losing out* on tasting that wonderful chocolate-chip cookie. Does that sound familiar? Many people are faced with that type of challenge – some on a daily basis.

Losing is not fun. Have you ever lost money? THAT really was stressful! Remember being lost on an unfamiliar road? Really a horrible feeling, wasn't it? How many of you have lost a game that you really wanted to win? We **lose** car keys, friends, valuable papers ... I could go on and on. Our lives are full of losses, some unavoidable. In our culture, losing is a negative verb which projects **great value** to the word that follows it. Think about it. It's truly ironic that we expect our brain to shift from the commonly shared meaning of **lose** and avoiding **loss** to **"TRYING TO LOSE" ... WEIGHT**. It is unreasonable to make negative suggestions to the brain, and still expect positive results. **What we say to ourselves – the internal language we use - is important, because it directly affects our attitude about eating.** Success in getting control over your weight, and maintaining it depends on a "winning" mindset rather than a "losing" mentality. **A winning mindset is the most positive state you can enjoy. It defines success and victory as you overcome obstacles, and draw upon your knowledge, your positive energy and motivation as well as your courage and commitment. You feel like a winner when you achieve your goals.**

Background

The battle lines are drawn against the expanding waistline. It's no wonder! There is an explosion of fast food restaurants around every corner, ready, willing and able to "supersize" you. Donut shops, ice cream stores, bagel and pastry outlets promote sweet treats; and even coffee emporiums offer "tall, grande, and venti" sizes of calorie-rich drinks. Manufacturers create colorful packaging and cute characters to market sweet foods, making them particularly attractive to children. Think about Fruit Loops "Toucan", the "Silly Rabbit" of Trix fame, or the Lucky Charms "Leprechaun" to name just a few. Advertisements in the print media and product placement on TV shows scream at us with all the power of imagery, enthusiasm, and words to influence our desire to eat their products. The same magazines that hype the latest "celebrity" diet also highlight pictures and recipes for high calorie, scrumptious, mouth-watering desserts.

It's hard when you can't even button your slacks without lying on the bed, and sucking up your stomach – then the buttons pop! It's not even necessary to be obese, to be engaged in a personal struggle to achieve your desired weight and clothing size. For all those who have "been there, done that", you know what I mean. It's easy to generate all the best intentions. It seems like a no-brainer because you can feel and see the effects of weighing more than you want, but you feel stuck in old habits. You've made all those New Year's Resolutions—time and time again. The determination and resolve works for about two to three days. Then, without any warning, the temptations take over once again. They seem small at first, but as they amass, these temptations seem to develop a life and intensity of their own.

Perhaps you have been waging this weight war from childhood, or maybe the "battle of *your* bulge" originated during a pregnancy, remained with you, and grew right along with your child. It's possible to think about what you are going to have for your next meal not more than ten minutes after the last one has been finished. Are you working hard to stay on diet plans that you thought would be helpful, but are constantly being tempted and distracted away from all those good intentions?

Temptations

Someone brings a box of doughnuts into the office; or you go by the Cinnabon kiosk at the mall. Oh my! They look so mouth-watering, and smell so-o good! Everyone who is anyone at the office is getting together at the nearby 'watering hole' to celebrate a promotion or achieving the latest contract coup. How can you refuse without seeming to be a party pooper? Another dilemma comes up when you are invited to dinner by your mother-in-law, your boss, boss's wife (or any other time where you really believe you can't say "No thank you"). It's very hard to refuse that specialty dinner of fried chicken, corn on the cob, mashed potatoes, hot homemade bread, and chocolate soufflé from a closely-guarded, secret family recipe, without generating hurt feelings? These are only a *few* of the forces that pull you away from all your good intentions and commitments. If you have become so discouraged that you have given up on yourself, this war seems like a "losing" battle. We all cannot help but wonder if we have the right weapons, adequate armor, appropriate strategies and tactics to actually *win* this war.

Purpose for the book

The good news is that you are not alone. These scenarios are widespread and common. My purpose in writing this book is to transform or change your relationship with food from one of limitation to that of empowerment. The difference between success and failure in getting and maintaining control over weight is a winning mindset rather than a losing mentality. Time-honored, successful, psychological strategies will reenergize your commitment to overcome the emotional conflicts and sabotages that have plagued you over a lifetime of struggle. It's well known that diets alone are ineffective in helping overweight people change what they weigh without finding other ways of satisfying emotional needs beyond putting food in their mouth.

Every good battle plan includes an assessment of your assets as well as an analysis of your needs to discover the skills, expertise, systematic approach, or information that you will need to develop in order to limit your liabilities. Any good general will also tell you to "know your enemy." In the weight war, this means giving labels to your temptations. Objectively evaluating the elements that detract you and pull you away from achieving victory will allow effective planning and help you to develop effective strategies. It is a change of lifestyle rather than a dedication to a specific diet.

One of my missions in life is to share successful, practical weight management strategies with as many people as possible. This is *not* a diet book, although there are many suggestions as to the best way to stay on any diet you choose. It is not a book on physical fitness, although a chapter on exercising by Kip Jawish gives you great ideas about including exercise and fitness into your daily routine. It is also not a cookbook, although there are some neat recipes and cooking techniques offered by my colleague, Jane Mercado, to help you adopt your desired lifestyle changes. The core of this book examines the structure of the most successful eating strategies, which will help you change your perspectives about food, as well as retrieve or create whatever emotional resources that are needed to make those approaches possible. I want to be your "general" to help you use relevant and appropriate strategies to win your war against excess weight.

Role of NLP

From as early as 1981 when I attended my first training in clinical hypnosis at the American Hypnosis Training Academy in Silver Spring, Maryland, I have been working to help clients transform their perspectives negative impacts on their lives. My clinical hypnosis practice is based on the work of Dr Milton H. Erickson; and **Neuro-Linguistic Programming** (NLP). NLP was developed by Richard Bandler and John Grinder in the 1970's. It is modeled on the mastery of three recognized experts in psychotherapy. **Milton H. Erickson, M.D.** is widely considered to be the 'father' of modern clinical hypnosis; **Virginia Satir, LCSW** was one of the leading family therapists who advocated for the value of 'family systems' in therapy, and the whole issue of 'self-esteem'. The third major therapist whose work is incorporated into NLP was **Fritz Perls, MD**, the creator of 'Gestalt Therapy'. The heart of Gestalt Therapy is the awareness of the union of feelings and behaviors in any context; and the connection between the 'self' and the outside world in the interest of fulfilling one's 'human potential'.

NLP identifies and uses the specific needs and unique internal resources of each person along with adopting more effective strategies to help them make the changes they want. "Neuro" relates to the input of your brain and nervous system. "Linguistic" refers to the language we use to interpret our experiences, the world and the ongoing self-talk. "Programming" is about understanding how our behavior is influenced by our internal experience and beliefs. The major philosophical perspectives that I have adopted to help people overcome the temptations and emotional sabotages which interfere with their success are based on the following selected assumptions promoted by NLP:

→ Behind every behavior there is a positive intention. When you can separate the negative effects of the behavior from the positive intention, or internal need which drives any unwanted behavior, you can find more efficient ways of satisfying that intention or need.

→ People already have all the internal resources they need to solve the problem about which they are complaining. Difficulties arise only if you are not aware that you possess that resource or if you don't know how to use it in the needed situation.

→ There is no failure, only feedback about what you can do differently to create different results.

→ The positive worth of an individual is undeniable. What **is** in question is the value and appropriateness of the selected behavior.

→ People make the best choices they can, with the resources they have at the time and the factors that might be influencing the situation.

You all may have heard (or used) the phrase, "A part of me wants to do 'X', while another part of me really wants to do 'Y'." whether it is to eat a salad versus eating a steak. Virginia Satir contributed the concept that one's emotional self is made up of many parts, all of whom are driven by psychological needs. When you identify these parts and the needs they attempt to serve on your behalf, you have the opportunities to meet the needs of each part appropriately, with the goal of resolving internal conflict. This is true even when the behaviors have negative consequences, such as overeating or eating fattening foods.

My training and work in NLP has given me the opportunity to learn effective techniques and strategies in changing internal emotional states which influence behavior. I have drawn heavily on the principles, philosophy, and techniques of these disciplines to help clients create effective strategies to accomplish their goals and to transform any limiting beliefs into empowering ones of excellence. This is particularly relevant to changing negative self-talk and limiting beliefs which sabotage your good intentions of achieving your goal weight.

All successes and victories require the recognition of a *specific* desired outcome. Just saying "I really want to lose some weight" will likely derail you from accomplishing anything because it is vague and unspecified. It is also disempowering since that phrase does not demand any specific action or behavior from you, regardless of the number of times you repeat it to yourself. It's hard to track your progress, much less know when to declare victory!

A Personal Story

I am also one of those women who have struggled with having gained excess weight, particularly after each of my three pregnancies. I put weight on very easily, especially around the waist and backside. Ironically, my wrists and ankles stayed thin, so if I wore loose clothes, many people didn't notice fluctuation in my weight. But *I* certainly noticed when my skirts and slacks didn't button around the waist. I had to develop a new strategy and philosophy about my eating and exercise habits. Over the nearly thirty years that I have been in a private, clinical practice, treating the various problems that motivate clients to seek counseling, I am struck by the frequency with which weight issues are either one of the main complaints, or aggravate the other presented problems.

The concept of *Win the Weight War* arose out of helping clients solve their particular weight struggles. The chapters attempt to address these concerns, and are full of specific examples of client stories and how each person worked through their struggles to win their personal war on weight. Each chapter explores one step in the process that teaches effective techniques to all those who feel stuck in their effort to achieve their weight goals. It's important to add that there is no rigid, lockstep strategy that determines how I work with clients on weight issues. As you will see, each person has separate stories, unique backgrounds, as well as different goals and needs. The strategies and interventions that are described here are those that have worked successfully for many people. It is my hope that they are expressed with enough clarity that anyone can use them for themselves. If you find you have additional stumbling blocks, limiting belief systems, or impasses that interfere with winning this weight war, you may choose to consult with a therapist to help you work through them.

Eating habits must be shifted over a lifetime. It is very different than stopping such destructive habits as smoking or drinking, which can be compared to an on/off switch on a lamp. If you make a commitment to never again engage in **those** habits, you will continue to live comfortably, if not healthier. Eating, on the other hand, is a necessity of life. Food is the fuel on which your body depends for survival. You will literally die of starvation if you stop eating altogether. Eating too much food will also cause physical distress and health dangers. If you think of a "dimmer switch" to modify your eating habits, you will enhance your health and remain in control of your weight. Sometimes decisions on what and how much to eat, are made as many as six times a day. It is vital to learn what you *can* eat—and to enjoy it thoroughly!

To that end, this book will focus on accessing your internal resources of your head, your heart and your "gut level" feeling of what you want, and what you are willing to do to get it.

→ **From your rational and logical part (your head),** you determine your **realistic** goal weight. What size will you be wearing? What will be the reactions of important people in your life? What are the "powerful' temptations in your life which pull you away from succeeding?

→ **From your heart,** what's **"in it"** for you to be at your goal weight? Focusing on getting these benefits and advantages for you will help you understand the **value and importance** of winning your war against overweight.

→ **From your guts,** Find the **courage or intestinal fortitude** to be in control of what kinds and how much food to put into your mouth, as well as how fast and how often you eat. Increasing the frequency, intensity, and duration of exercise causes your metabolism to burn up more calories

The Underlying Factors

Win the Weight War examines the factors that can cause weight problems, the emotional needs that food attempts to satisfy, as well as identifying those sabotages that prevent you from reducing that weight, and how to overcome them. The principles included here are designed to help you redefine your "love affair" with food by identifying your weight goals, giving purpose and importance to achieving those goals, providing specific suggestions and strategies to build motivation, and helping you win *your* war on weight.

The major factors explored here to help you be successful in winning your personal weight war are:

- → Setting a realistic goal with appropriate milestones to evaluate progress.

- → Making a positive statement about what you want, and focusing on the future, so your brain will concentrate on the achievement of that success rather than obsess about all the times in the past that you tried and failed.

- → Motivation: What's in it for you to be at your goal weight? The health benefits of staying slender are very well known, yet they rarely motivate anyone to change anything, much less ingrained eating habits.

- → You want to be "sweet" to yourself by honoring your values and move closer to your important goals.

- → Create within yourself an ally and cheerleader who will *remind* you of the benefits of winning your personal battles with weight, and encourage you to keep focused on your goal.

- → Quality of food: How do you decide what to put into your mouth, as well as how you choose how much food that you choose to eat?

- → Rate of food consumption, and the frequency with which you eat. Slowing down, and eating less food more often

- → The psychological and emotional needs and the 'positive intentions' that drive those overeating behaviors and seem to sabotage your best intentions and commitment

- → Resolving internal conflicts, which can sabotage your best intentions

→ Transforming the limiting belief systems into more empowering ones

→ The frequency, intensity and duration of exercise

→ Staying in control when you eat out

→ Selection and preparation of food to maximize taste and minimize calories

These treatment philosophies form the basis for the strategies and interventions that clients have found to be very successful and effective over the years. They transform how you:

→ Decide what is important to you about setting your desired weight, and maintaining it

→ Choose the food you eat.

→ Decide how much to eat.

→ Determine the pace and frequency of eating.

→ Determine how frequently and intensely you exercise.

→ Satisfy any emotional needs associated with your eating behavior.

Chapters Overview

A brief overview of the chapters might help you understand the organization of this *Win the Weight War* book.

In Chapter One, we will explore how struggles with weight have reached a crisis in America. The factors discussed are physiological, psychological, genetic, gender, sedentary lifestyles, economic limitations, addictions, emotional connections to food or are just habit related

Creating a compelling outcome that actually *works* is the focus of the second chapter. The rationale is that the outcome needs to be *so* important to your well-being that it's worth the effort it will take. This is the one success factor that is most often missing in one's resolutions, vows, or promises. It's exciting to watch people get enthused about formulating a plan of action. The most frequent comment heard is "Finally, I feel like I'm on my way!"

The third chapter discusses how words matter to ones unconscious awareness which actually motivates our actions. You will understand why the concept of "losing" weight is a negative motivator. Our culture teaches us to avoid losses since they imply that we will be deprived of something important in our lives. You want to transform a "losing" mindset into a "winning" mentality.

Chapter Four helps you create your own personal cheerleader which means that you will have a powerful ally in your struggle. An actual transcript of the process is included giving a vivid example of how to generate this powerful resource.

Foot-soldiers in this weight war often complain that they don't have a consistent way of determining when they are hungry, or, above all, knowing when to *stop* eating. Many overweight people only stop eating when their stomachs are full.

The title of the fifth chapter is "Internal Signal Corps: A Fistfull of Food Will Fill You". This chapter offers a successful strategy to get in control of how much you eat, by developing an acute awareness of the sensations in your stomach. You will stop eating when you feel comfortable, rather than full or stuffed.

The sixth chapter helps you to slow down the rate and frequency with which you eat, allowing you to enjoy every bite to its fullest potential. When you thoroughly enjoy the taste of the food you eat, you will no longer feel deprived or discouraged.

Chapter Seven is essential in the success of this battle by exploring the kinds of sabotages and temptations which pull you away from your commitment to your goal. Some of these sabotages are formed from internal conflicts which pit getting to your goal weight with the effort that it will take to achieve it. Choices of successful alternatives are offered to conquer these sabotages because each person is unique in terms of which and how those sabotages are impactful.

In the next chapter, Chapter Eight, we specifically explore how to fight the "Battle of Emotional Hunger". Because most people claim they overeat when they are stressed, feel upset, anxious, or discouraged, once they find better ways to handle this stress, they feel empowered and confident. You will learn to create and use positive internal resources to protect you from these negative forces in your life.

Chapter Nine focuses on the role of physical fitness in your weight management program and was co-authored by Kip Jawish, a personal fitness trainer, who created In-Fit Fitness Studio in Frederick Maryland. The value of working with a personal trainer is discussed, but exploring all the informal ways that you can have fun including exercise in your life, is even more important.

Eating out in restaurants has always been a challenge until now. Chapter Ten offers practical tips and guidelines to reassure you that you can enjoy all the social benefits of eating out while honoring your commitment to yourself and achieving your goal weight.

Do you *love* to cook? Is it not only a hobby, but a calling? On the other hand, is it a passion that seems to sabotage your best intentions? You certainly don't want to give up that hobby—and you don't have to! Jane Mercado, MA, Licensed Clinical Professional Counselor, and a longtime colleague has been a successful and healthy winner of her personal weight war. She has developed wonderful food selection and cooking strategies that can work to transform any of your favorite recipes from "fat-full" to fabulous, while maintaining all the good flavor and consistency that made them your favorites. She co-authored the eleventh chapter entitled "Winning the Cooking Game."

The last chapter is the conclusion, summarizing the main points of the book alphabetically. It's a fun way to review and remember the main points.

For simplicity in writing, I have written this book as if you were sitting across from me in counseling or in a coaching context, with lots of examples to illustrate points. To avoid confusion, third person pronouns are consistently written as "she," unless I am referring specifically to a male client. The suggestions are certainly applicable to everyone. The names and/or specific identifying details cited in client case studies have been changed to preserve privacy.

I am not a nutritionist or food specialist. There are plenty of wonderful resources of cookbooks and diet plans that specialize in analyzing diets and eating habits. Effective nutritional eating programs such as Weight Watchers, and those run by hospitals and wellness centers both in the United States and in many other countries will actually teach you to make appropriate nutritional decisions. I am an equal opportunity advocate for all structured diet plans. *They will all work—if you stay committed to any one of them.* As one of my clients said, somewhat plaintively, "The hardest thing about staying on a diet is…*staying* on the diet." Many have expressed their preferences, varying from devotees of Weight Watchers, Atkins, South Beach, or even Scarsdale. They just don't *stick* with any of them! I want to help you build powerful motivations so that you stay committed to whatever structure of weight management you prefer.

It is really important for you to get a thorough physical examination by a physician who knows you well. He or she can make sure that your problems with weight are caused by unhealthy eating habits and strategies and not a physical ailment or metabolic problem that manifests as weight gain. .

If you do not want to make positive changes in your body shape, size or weight, this book is not for you.

CHAPTER 1

"Heavy" Encounters: The Reality Check

Everyone has an inborn, important relationship with food. It is essential to maintaining life from the very moment we are born. Our bodies transform or metabolize what we eat into necessary energy and nutrients. Our ability to function deteriorates without enough nutritious food. Starvation like the type experienced by the "living skeletons" in poverty-stricken countries or by the victims of atrocities in the Nazi concentration camps, attests to the fact that without food, *we will die.* Of course, if we eat *too* much, we run the risk of dying from the complications of obesity. In the immortal words of "Roseanne Roseanna-Danna," so aptly portrayed by Gilda Radner on *Saturday Night Live*: **"It's always something!"**

Obesity, or being significantly overweight, is one of the biggest health issues in America. To state the obvious, it results from an imbalance of food intake and energy output—or taking in and storing more calories than are burned up. One pound of body weight is estimated to contain 3,500 calories. Fat (or adipose) cells form at birth, and like sponges, they absorb or release stored up fat. These cells are generally found under the skin and in soft tissue around our internal organs. The bottom line is that if a person's weight is over 20 percent of their ideal weight, they are considered obese. The dangers of being overweight are well known. Health statistics reflect the medical concerns about diabetes, high cholesterol, stroke risk, as well as causing high blood pressure, requiring the heart to pump harder. For example, BarnesCare, a large non-profit healthcare organization, explores the increase in health care costs and the loss of productivity generated by obesity in an article,

"Controlling Obesity in the Workplace". It quotes a study from the US Department of Health and Human Services stating that 129 million Americans are overweight or obese. DHHS further estimates that the economic costs of being overweight vary from $69 billion to $117 billion dollars.

Factors Affecting Weight

There are many complex factors that affect what we weigh, and how easily or quickly we gain or reduce that weight. We ignore the physiological and biochemical factors, illnesses and injuries, or genetics at our own peril.

The selection of a sedentary career or lifestyle, as well as the onset of pregnancy, menopause, and other hormonal changes will affect what you weigh. Even addictive behaviors are factors in adding pounds. It's also possible that emotional links to food or just bad eating habits, contribute to overweight.

Physiological and Biochemical Factors

Our personal metabolisms change with such things as the selection of a sedentary career, inactive lifestyle, pregnancy, menopause, or other hormonal changes. As we age, our bodies no longer require the same amount of food or number of calories to be efficiently nourished. Therefore, even when we eat a balanced diet in moderation, the chances are that we will still gain weight as we get older. It's not accidental that many restaurants offer menus for senior citizens with smaller portions (not to mention lower prices). It is essential that in order to manage our weight successfully, we learn to adapt our lifestyles and eating habits to these changing physiological requirements.

According to Dr. Craig Freudenrich, all of our fat cells are present at our birth. He describes them as being like tiny plastic bags that fill up with, and stores fatty acids. Fat has positive uses in terms of "metabolizing energy, heat insulation and mechanical cushioning". Fat cells tend to capture glucose and amino acids, which have been absorbed into the bloodstream after a meal and convert these into fat molecules stored in these tiny bags. Your body chemistry converts fatty acid into fat cells **much** more efficiently than proteins or complex carbohydrates that require **ten** times more energy to make this transformation possible. When you are exercising, or at the very least refraining from eating food, your body pulls on the internal stored energy, formed by breaking down carbohydrates. "Your weight is determined by the rate at which you store energy from the food you eat, and the rate at which you use that energy. Remember that as your body breaks down the fat, the number of fat cells remain the same; each fat cell simply gets smaller."

Addictions

Addictions must be included as a factor in weight problems. Alcohol abuse is an obvious one. Beer, wine, or liquors are full of empty calories from sugars. Alcohol and drug addiction studies support the contention that addictions change the biochemistry of our bodies. Many would argue that body chemistry undergoes similar changes in response to sugars, creating an intense physical urge for additional high caloric foods that are rich in sugars. It is often easier to say "no" *before* we consume a sweet than it is to attempt to stop eating it once we have begun. In support of this food addiction theory, some people develop a panic response about limiting the quantity of food they consume, believing that they will starve.

Gender

Gender is an important factor in our consideration of individual eating habits. Many women complain that they eat the very same things as their husbands, yet they add on weight, while their partners seem to maintain their weight consistently. Men tend to have a higher resting metabolic rate than women do, implying that they require more calories to maintain their body weight than a woman of similar bone structure and size. Since men don't generally go through intense hormonal shifts such as pregnancy or menopause, their hormones tend to be more stable than those of women.

Men and women also store fat inn different parts of their bodies. Many men tend to gain weight around the belly which prevents slacks from fitting properly. It often results in a sloppy, unkempt appearance. Many women tend to gain weight around the hips, buttocks, and thighs, as well as the waist, which can even out the distribution, hiding the appearance of the weight more effectively. Some women also put weight on as a protective layer to keep them safe from unwanted sexual advances.

Illnesses and injuries

Physical disabilities or difficulties are certainly important factors in contributing to obesity. They affect how we *can* exercise, and often reduce our motivation to exercise vigorously on a regular basis. Illnesses also affect how easily we can digest foods, and sometimes, the kinds of foods we are allowed to eat. Medications often have side effects that impact how we metabolize food and how energetic we feel. When we feel physically ill, hurt, vulnerable, nervous, or frightened, the need for comfort increases dramatically. Since eating has represented comfort from our earliest memories as small children we tend to choose those foods that are highest in calories and carbohydrates to help comfort us when we are feeling pain and discomfort.

Sedentary lifestyles

Inactivity is a socially acceptable lifestyle, evidenced by our unwillingness to even get up from the couch to change the channels on TV. We use the remote. These habits of inactivity result in exercise becoming a chore and a challenge. Our distant ancestors never had to worry about being overweight. Just to survive, they expended more energy and calories than they consumed. Work was rigorous and seemingly constant. No additional exercise was necessary. As technology and science created labor-saving machines, surviving in a contemporary culture meant developing specialized abilities. Modern men and women focus on using their brains to earn a living rather than their bodies.

Since so many Americans tend to sit at computers, watch TV or get away in their cars on weekends instead of physically exerting themselves, they add more weight than during the week according to an article by Susan Racette. Additional muscular exertion is needed to maintain the metabolic efficiency to keep bodies healthy and fit.

It has become even tougher for many children who don't get as much exercise as previous generations did. Instead of being encouraged to "go outside and play," kids will chill out in front of their video games, computers, or television sets. For many, there is no safe place to play outside. Not everyone lives where there is green grass, a yard, or a playground nearby. Unfortunately, many school systems have responded to budget cuts by reducing the requirements for physical fitness courses. Intramural sports and activities inside the school day have been cut for the same reasons. In response to the national drive to enhance academic achievement, elementary schools have even reduced the amount of time children spend running around during recess. If public schools offered planned after-school physical activities, it would kill two birds with one stone. Not only would it reduce the amount of time spent by "latch-key" kids watching TV at home, but it would give them supervised, aerobic activities that would burn off excess calories, develop good exercise habits, and build strong bones and muscles.

Psychological Factors

Most eating behaviors are learned from the early examples, and/or life-style choices set for us by caretakers. Since our very existence depends on being nourished with food, eating is the first behavior we learn. We are completely dependent on caregivers to supply food, which others prepare. Food represents comfort, nurturance, and an intimate connection with the person providing this nourishment. We are not capable of evaluating our nutrition choices effectively. As children, even if we had sufficient education and information about proper nutrition, we would not have had the capacity, maturity, money or experience to put it into practice. We could not control the quantities of food or the amounts of fat and sugar that we were given.

The psychological repercussions of not trusting our own bodies to know when we have had enough to eat are reflected in a long-term inability to know when to *stop* eating. There is also a tendency for children to rebel against eating demands by parents. One of the many complex factors which create eating disorders is born in response to wanting independence from demands or the implicit pressure to be perfect. These disorders include compulsive, habitual overeating (or binging), which leads to obesity, or the equally compulsive fear of gaining weight (anorexia); as well as binging, then purging by inducing vomiting or abusing laxatives (bulimia).

Emotions continue to play a major role in the motivation for overeating. When we become anxious, depressed, angry, hurt or upset, our eating habits are affected. We revert back to the earliest recognizable means of comfort. We eat! Eating becomes compulsive when we focus on what we believe to be our intrinsic losses, or feel less than competent to cope with the challenges that face us. We will explore this in greater length in Chapter Eight.

Economic Factors

Economics factors are important in maintaining overweight lifestyles as foods that are both affordable and plentiful tend to be high in simple carbohydrates and fats. If one eats large quantities in an effort to stave off the fears of hunger or deprivation, one would not necessarily be assured of where the next meal would be coming from. Eating healthy vegetables and lean meats cost more than many families can afford to spend on their food budget, particularly with the costs of housing, heating oil, electricity, and gasoline climbing precariously. On the other hand, obesity results in more complicated medical problems and even higher medical costs for treatment.

Socio-cultural Factors

We are influenced by family expectations and cultures. In some traditional cultures, one is not considered well off, unless or until one is "well fed." A "good" wife is sometimes defined by how well she cooks, as evidenced by the girth of her family members.

The values of the "clean plate club" and "not wasting food when people are starving in Africa (or India)" were handed down from the generation who lived through and survived the "Great Depression" and the necessary sacrifices of the Second World War. This mentality was born out of the necessity to cope with the deprivation of food shortages, widespread poverty and the inability of a great many people to work; much less to earn a living wage. The concept, "You can't leave this table until you have finished your food," means well, but is misguided. By doing so, we are implicitly telling children: "Don't trust the sensations your body is generating." Eating in a restaurant a few months ago, a friend and I watched a mother reprimand her young daughter for not finishing the hot dog in a bun and the French fries that were on her plate. The little girl had eaten half of the hot dog and some of the fries. The overweight mother was so angry that she threatened her child with a spanking if she did not finish her dinner. The slender little girl looked very distressed and ate the rest of the hot dog. The mother promptly grumbled at her daughter, and reached over to finish her fries. My friend sadly shook her head, and mentioned that the weight of the mother was beside the point. That scene reminded her of her own childhood when her own slender mother continually criticized her for leaving food on her plate.

Our American culture seems to struggle with complaints about widespread obesity as contrasted to the multiple magazines that highlight appetizing, delicious, high-calorie desserts along with the recipes for preparing them, as well as the huge number of high-calorie choices featured in food stores, restaurants, and even in vending machines, which are sometimes the only foods offered at many employee worksites. There are also the more subtle influences of product placement in movies and television shows.

Dieting is not the entire answer either. Even though it may help over the short term, it does not provide us with lifestyle changes which we can sustain over the long term. Plus, the word *diet* has a social connotation of denial and deprivation. We generally motivate ourselves to avoid deprivation of the things we want and like. If we change our understanding of the "*d*" word to indicate simply an objective *description* of the foods we eat, *whatever they are,* we can remain optimistic about including alternative foods in our diets that will nourish our bodies as well as satisfy our taste preferences.

Summary

This chapter explores the factors that impact and influence what we weigh and how, what, when and how much we eat. Our upbringing, expectations, emotional hardiness or vulnerability, and habits often contribute to our weight.

Food is essential to maintaining life. Unlike behaviors such as smoking cigarettes, using drugs or drinking alcohol, eating food is a necessity to preserving life. Therefore it's important to modify and control our intake of food so that it is in balance with the ways that we efficiently use the energy and nourishment that food is providing.

Unfortunately, the struggle with being overweight is literally one of the biggest health issues in America, resulting from taking in, and storing more calories than are burned up. Our personal metabolisms are often dependant on such things as the selection of a sedentary career, inactive lifestyle, pregnancy, menopause, or other hormonal changes. We must take into account the body and bone structure that we inherit. Our age and gender provide additional considerations, as our older bodies no longer require the same amount of food or number of calories to be efficiently they used to when our lifestyles were more active. Women have a different metabolism from men given the vastly different array of hormones.

The presence of illnesses and injuries might prevent or limit the degree or kind of exercise in which we can engage. We are influenced by family expectations and culture, not to mention traditional cooking styles, sometimes maintained to preserve ties to the family. Compulsive or binge eating can lead to obesity; as well as to the equally compulsive and physically dangerous disorders of anorexia and bulimia. Substance addictions are a wildcard factor in weight challenges as they often add empty calories and decrease available funds for nutritious foods. By bringing these factors into the forefront of our minds, we can begin to make appropriate and realistic choices about how we eat. To manage our weight, we must construct an imaginary "dimmer switch" to control our selection and portions of food, which is exactly what the following ten strategies will enable you to do. The first strategy focuses on setting yourself up for success by defining your outcome in a compelling way which pulls you into it.

CHAPTER 2

Strategy One: Create a Compelling Future

Have you ever wanted something so badly that you could "taste" it? It was so real that you could almost reach out and touch it. This makes the objective very clear and increases the likelihood that you will be victorious in winning it. You could certainly identify *exactly* what the aim was; therefore, you were easily able to determine if and when you had successfully achieved it. Being effectively motivated requires that you know what you want, can recognize it when you get it and are enthused about achieving it.

Elements of success

There are two required elements for success in setting and achieving your goals. The first is having enough factual information to help you to make *logical* decisions about how to structure your goals to make them doable. You also will want to identify the resources you need to be successful. The second is to identify the important values the goals represent, which can inspire and motivate you to do whatever it takes to achieve the goals you have set.

Goals are always future oriented. Focusing on the past is irrelevant, even though you may have achieved other outcomes. It removes motivation because they have already been achieved.

When you specify an outcome that you want to accomplish, you have the power to make it as vivid and desirable as you can. This outcome will generate its own compelling power to pull you into it. You then have ability to assess your values, personal strengths and resources objectively, as well as to evaluate the opposite forces of temptation, discouragement, or obstacles from the "dark side" that will pull you away from winning. Getting to *any* goal necessitates evaluating that this goal is worth the effort that it would take to overcome these barriers to achieving it. This is the part of the process that relates to the 'head'. It is the rational aspect of winning this weight war. You need all the positive rationales possible to add to your ammunition. Sometimes the rational part of you must take charge of the emotional drives which pull you away from your goals. Remember that winning the weight war is an ongoing, daily commitment to a long-term personal project.

Weight History

An exploration of your weight history will give you some insight into the issues that drive you to eat, and the beliefs about food that now influence your eating habits and behaviors. This may provide a roadmap of sorts to give you direction in resolving conflicts or confusion. Many clients can see the roots of their overeating habits and diminishing self-esteem represented in their childhood experiences.

The following questions will give you "food for thought":

Self-esteem and Weight

1. Did you have an awareness of your weight as a child?
2. As a child or an adolescent, were you ever teased about your weight?
3. Were many family members overweight?
4. What was the conventional wisdom in your family about food and eating as you grew up? For example, was there an inherent value in being a member of the "clean plate club"?
5. Were you made to stay at the table until *all* your "vegetables were eaten?"

6. Was having enough to eat an ongoing problem, or was abundant food spoiling or going to waste?

7. Has your social life ever been affected by your weight?

8. How does a five-pound increase (or decrease) in weight affect your self-confidence?

9. Are you presently involved in an occupation that requires or encourages you to maintain a certain weight?

As you give some thought to these questions, you may find that memories of feelings, events, or conversations clearly come to mind. It's also possible that many of these particular questions are not directly applicable to you. In that case, you may explore your best recollection of when and how your weight began to negatively impact you. The issues highlighted in this short questionnaire link your experiences with weight to how you value yourself or how you believe others respond to you.

Abigail:

Abigail was a forty-one-year-old, divorced administrative assistant, who spent her entire childhood being the butt of family jokes, and being called names such as "cow-butt" and "thunder-thighs." She reported that the harder she tried to reduce, and "be good" about eating the "right foods," the more the teasing escalated. Her parents were divorced. "Mother" had been busy keeping her current husband happy, and focused the bulk of her attention on her two young sons from the second marriage. There were multiple snacks available, although Abigail was roundly criticized for indulging in them. It was a double-edged sword in that she identified eating as her only com-

fort. Hearing her behavior criticized, and having it enabled by the adults in the family at the same time was a double bind, which increased her sense of confusion, shame, and unworthiness; and touched all parts of her life. As a result, she could not easily accept compliments or recognize positive accomplishments. It felt like whichever path she chose, she would be the object of criticism and disdain. This highlighted her need to disregard and dispute the validity of the family criticism. It was important for Abigail to put this criticism into an objective perspective that had less to do with her, and much more to do with the insensitivity and inconsiderate behavior of the people in her early life.

To add to the complexity of a dysfunctional family of origin, her first marriage was filled with unreasonable demands and physical abuse. Once Abigail left that relationship, she ate compulsively as a way of asserting her independence and providing protection from being emotionally vulnerable. She felt out of control as she put on more weight.

The more specific you make the outcomes you set for yourself, the more you will feel connected to them. It needs to *matter* whether or not you succeed. Contrast Abigail's concerns with those of Allison.

Allison:

Allison, a thirty-nine year-old mother of three children, two teenage daughters and a ten year-old son, and had put on pounds with each child. She had a loving relationship with her husband of twenty years. Difficulties arose when her 18- and 16-year-old daughters didn't bring their friends to the house (particularly the boyfriends). When confronted, they tearfully told their mother that they were embarrassed by her weight. That really shook Allison because the last thing she wanted was to embarrass and/or alienate her children. Even her husband admitted that he was concerned about the effects of the weight on her heart since heart disease ran in her family.

Allison made a decision to reduce her weight down to 135 pounds, which was the weight the doctor recommended for her build. She made a long list of all the possible benefits including her health, increased recreation opportunities, self respect, respect from her children, admiration from her husband and the privilege of wearing fashionable clothes that would look good on her. She discovered that once she identified all the possible advantages of being at her goal weight, she could better visualize herself enjoying those benefits. It was a new perspective for Allison as she realized that she had not focused on her ultimate weight outcome with the same effective attitude and mindset that she had used when she committed herself to a graduate school program, and succeeded in earning her master's degree.

Identify Personal Internal Resources

You will want to identify and make a connection with all your internal resources that are available to help you win those goals, (even those resources which you might have overlooked or disregarded). Remember to take into account all the important benefits that go along with achieving them so that you maintain your high motivation.

Being creative can produce options and alternatives that you may not have considered before. It allows us to think outside the proverbial box of all those failed attempts to solve the problems in the past. This is very important, since many people struggle with weight for long periods of time. Additionally, successful weight management does not always follow a linear path. Sometimes it's two steps forward and one step backward.

> *It was necessary for Allison to rethink her choices and options in imaginative and resourceful ways. She could experiment with the other strategies that we had discussed, without ascribing blame or shame for past difficulties or failures. After giving this a great deal of thought, Allison wrote down a list of possibilities, some of which were "tried and true" successful strategies, such as remembering her determination to graduate from college, and how she formed a study group to get through a particularly demanding course. She could connect with others at her gym to be "weight" partners. Others were creative fantasies about what she could do. Among these was making up a game in which she would score points every time she said "no thank you" and resisted the temptation to eat foods which contained high amounts of fat and calories. (She allowed bonus points when she resisted her favorite foods.) When she collected 100 points, she treated herself to a massage.*

The success of *any* strategy depends on how valuable the outcome is to you. That outcome has to be worth the effort that it will take to make it happen. Ask yourself the following questions to determine the *true worth* of your weight goal and how important it is to you:

Personal Values of Achieving Goal Weight

1. What are all the things that accomplishing my goal weight and maintaining it at that level will do for me, that are important, and are worth the effort it will take?

   Abigail discovered that she had to prove to herself that she could set a goal and achieve it for herself rather than as a reaction to pressure from others, whether positive or negative. It was the sense of her being in control of her decisions that made it so worthwhile. She would feel comfortable in clothes that were stylish. She would take personal pride in achieving a goal that had been elusive. There was a part of her that truly wanted to give those that teased (tortured) her, a well deserved come-uppance!

2. How will I behave differently than I do now, when I have reached my goal weight?

   Abigail imagined that she would stand straighter, walk and talk more confidently, as well as become assertive in standing up for herself with family members.

3. In your minds eye, imagine yourself as you are *right now*, as if you were looking at   yourself in a mirror, or as someone else would see you. How do you feel inside when you see that image?

   "I am very unhappy, frustrated, and angry when I look at myself in the mirror every morning. I

*think my friends and family look down on me. I feel
disrespected, no matter how accommodating and nice
I try to be."*

4. Does that image feel familiar or alienated?

*"It's as if the person who lives inside of me weighs
only 120 pounds, rather than the 180-pound person
that I know exists in reality, and in the "mirror" of
my mind's eye. I am always a little shocked when I
walk past a store window, and see my reflection in
the mirror. I get depressed when I realize that it is
me after all."*

*Abigail was very surprised at the intensity of
her emotional response to these questions.*

5. Have there been any benefits or "gains" that have accompanied
   your present weight? That is, what would you miss by being
   at your goal weight?

*"The longer I thought about it the more sense
it made to think about benefits of my weight. The
extra weight was just a plausible excuse to explain
why I didn't have a boyfriend. After all, men would
not really be interested or attracted to me when I am
heavy. I don't want to go through the emotional stress
ever again."*

*Abigail recognized that the weight actually
served to protect her from being emotionally or physically hurt. We discussed how she might honor and preserve this positive intention. She decided that a better
way of protecting herself was to be very particular
about the quality of men that she could meet. Since*

alcohol abuse had been a theme in her family, she decided she didn't want to visit bars. After making a list of possible resources, Abigail joined the local YMCA where there were many opportunities to exercise – as well as having the advantage of attracting men who shared the interest of fitness. A non-credit class in computer technology offered necessary career skills as well as a non-threatening environment to meet people. As she continued to work through the psychological issues surrounding her childhood, she even understood that since she no longer needed emotional approval from her family back when she was a child, she could make her own food decisions.

There may be comforting or important elements about keeping **your** present weight that are subtle, and which might be in conflict with your other values. For example, budgeting for new clothes at smaller sizes may be an economic nightmare. Having kids angrily complain, or throw tantrums because their favorite snack foods are no longer available might be bitter pills to swallow in the interests of winning your battles over excess weight; and possibly save them from that fate.

6. Can you identify anything in your personal experience that would prevent you from accomplishing your goal?

Looking at the temptation or sabotage factors that could keep you from achieving what you want will arm you to take preventive action. The antidote to these roadblocks is to remember the important values wrapped up in getting to your goals. Stay *calm*, and connect with your experiences of competence, which maintain motivation and inspiration, even when circumstances seem to be sabotaging your success. When you make your goals and outcomes *concrete*, you ensure that they are easily defined and that the means to achieving them is recognizable. You can stay aware and mindful of what the effort is all worth to you. If your goals stay abstract, you give yourself psychological "wriggle room" or the opportunity to "cop out."

Abigail was very concerned that her eating habits had been ingrained, and her early learned behavior would outlast all her good intentions. She was worried that she would miss the tastes and foods that she loved, even though she understood the benefits of being slender. It was a temptation she was sure would derail all her healthy intentions.

For another example of this concept:

Alexis:

Alexis, on the other hand, grew up in a family where all the women (and most of the men) were highly overweight. For as long as anyone could recall, her family shared both sad and happy occasions with get-togethers including great feasts to which everyone contributed food, conversation, as well as comfort. Unfortunately, Alexis believed that if she changed her weight appreciably, she might be seen as being snobby or arrogant because she would not be eating the same high-carbohydrate, high-fat foods that were part-and-parcel of her family tradition. She didn't want to lose this strong emotional connection that had been so important to her. She was afraid there would be an emotional price to be paid if she were successful in reducing her weight. Her slender cousin was made fun of and "shunned" from family get-togethers. Alexis believed that her extra weight was a testament to her commitment to keeping her family's Italian cooking traditions alive. It was a real struggle for her to define what she wanted for herself.

Another problem arose when glitches occurred in her life. Alexis would become easily frustrated, overwhelmed, and often felt incompetent. Eating was her habitual way to feel security. To change this, I asked Alexis to recall experiences in her life when she had handled events calmly and competently. It was easier to put these temporary frustrations into their proper perspective and to focus on her real goals.

The Four C's: Commitment, Consistency, Control, Confidence.

Some other necessities of designing a compelling future can be thought of as the four *C*s:

1. ***Commitment*** to goals. Most people literally and figuratively experience an internal sensation of determination and discipline that allows them to know they are taking themselves seriously.

   Alexis revealed that the reason she had not been successful in the past was that she had given "lip service" to the issue of controlling her weight, and had not taken herself seriously.

2. **Consistency** relates to the ability to make a habit of engaging in behaviors that are different from the negative eating habits of the past. The strategies must be used regularly and continually, so they become automatic. They will feel very natural if given enough practice and reassurance that they are helpful and healthy habits. Consider that it generally takes three weeks for a behavior to begin to feel like a habit

Alexis recognized that if she continued to eat the way she had learned in her childhood, she would continue to weigh much more than she wanted. She needed to develop new decisions and strategies about choosing which healthy foods to eat, and how much of them to eat, so that healthy lifestyle becomes a habit.

3. **Control** acknowledges that you have the ultimate decision and choice of the kinds of food you eat, when, and how often you eat, as well as how much food you put into your mouth. Control is a habit and quality that most people identify as being important in their lives, yet it seems to be the first one to disappear when they get stressed. Control over eating relates to making continual evaluations as to the importance of eating a specific kind of food compared to enjoying the benefits of getting to your goal weight.

After some discussion on the issue of how she could stay in "consistent" control of her food choices, Alexis determined that she needed more physical and emotional support for these changes. She joined Weight Watchers, and was pleased with their system of helping her be in control of her what and how she ate.

4. *Confidence* is the fourth element of a compelling future as it reinforces your faith and ability to have the appropriate knowledge and resources to make your desired future relevant and real for you. It usually connects with a sense of excitement and positive expectation.

Alexis reported that as she developed additional confidence in her ability to actually do what was required to get the changes she wanted, the diet structure she adopted became easier to maintain.

Negativity

You are pulled away from these elements of adequate confidence, control, consistency and commitment by such negative emotions as fear, doubt, discouragement, and impatience. A lack of clarity, inconsistency, bad habits and exhaustion interfere with the commitment to achieving the goals. They are the sabotages that are even more important than specific food temptations. You fail to achieve your goals when you make the obstacles that seem to stand in your way, appear larger, more important, and more concrete than the objectives and goals you have set. Learning to overcome these factors is an important skill in winning the weight war. Write down these negative messages as you hear them in your mind, so you can evaluate them objectively. How relevant are these messages in the present, regardless of the value they had in the past?

Success Mind-set

Success is a state of mind, although the specific criteria will vary depending on the values of each person. What one person might consider as evidence of success, another might regard as a failure. *Webster's Encyclopedic Unabridged Dictionary of the English Language* defines success as ***"The favorable or prosperous termination of attempts or endeavors."*** Henry David Thoreau offers another take on the definition: ***"Success is when we are confidently advancing in the directions of our dreams".***

I invite each of you to consider success in the weight war as an ongoing experience—a 'process' rather than just an event that ends suddenly. The only way you can measure success is to chart your progress in quantifiable, small measures in which you can take pride. As Marcus Aurelius advised, ***"Go forward as occasion offers. Never look around to see whether any shall note it. Be satisfied with success in even the smallest matter, and think that even such a result is no trifle."*** That is the essence of keeping yourself motivated and enthused about staying on your journey toward the outcome you have specified. Maintaining your goal weight is the life long challenge which requires life-style changes rather than "dieting."

Think of Norman Vincent Peale, and his book *The Power of Positive Thinking*. A dominating dream and intense desire pave the way for successful achievement such that our inner strength and full commitment is focused on turning it into reality. Accomplishing those outcomes has to be so important to you that it is worth the effort that it takes.

The Mental Rehearsal for Self-esteem Exercise

This is designed to use your most powerful internal resources by comparing a created internal image of your most desirable future to a recollection of your most positive experience of undeniable success. For instance, remember a time when you needed determination, courage, and persistence to overcome those challenges or roadblocks that stood in your way. The pride that you experienced when you succeeded in the past, is the very drive and power that you will need to achieve victory in this struggle. It is included in its entirety in Appendix III.

Making a Strong Commitment

This is the part of the process which originates from the guts. Having the courage to follow through on what you want and what you have determined you will get for yourself. Setting up a strong commitment to making desired changes in attitude, perspective and beliefs is one of the most effective techniques to accomplish those goals. The steps to establishing this commitment are simple—and a few would say, easy. Most find this to be the most challenging part of winning your personal battle of the bulge. Since this thought process is different from the ordinary way of describing what one wants, it takes a conscious effort and some practice to make it happen.

➥ Start with a **realistic evaluation** of where you are at the present time. It seems almost too obvious to mention that the very act of reading this book on how to win your battle with weight indicates a desire to change the present state.

➥ The next step is to create a new visual image of a realistic, desirable future that will be **so attractive and compelling**, that you will be pulled into it. It's then possible to focus on what you need to successfully make that change. There is no accomplishment without a dream to spur it on. Martin Luther King underscored this philosophy with his "I have a dream" speech, which inspired millions to identify with the socio-political outcome he envisioned for the nation. New laws were passed and attitudes were transformed.

➥ The main caution is that this dream or desired outcome needs to be based on realistic goals and objectives, so that all the relevant considerations, potential concerns, or drawbacks are taken into account. It would be improbable and discouraging to plan on dropping over fifty pounds in a specific time such as three or six months in order to fit into a wedding dress.

The following is adapted from the American Hypnosis Training Academy, and provides a model of how to successfully create a compelling future.

Compelling Outcome

In order to have the best chance of achieving success, a goal must be:

1. Stated in Positive Language.

Negative statements contradict the importance of the behavior or change and only focus on achieving what you don't want. Consider the demand, "Don't think of Mickey Mouse or Minnie Mouse." In order to process that request or demand, our neurology requires that you conceptualize those two images. Then you can't "not" think of them. As another example, have you ever had a song or a part of a song run through your mind, even though you did everything you could to avoid it? The more you program our minds to formulate specific plans, the better equipped you will be to notice opportunities and respond appropriately so that our objectives are met. You can also realize when you are getting off track and can make appropriate corrections.

If you don't know where you are going, you won't know if you get there or not! One is reminded of Alice's adventures in Wonderland as she asks the Cheshire Cat:

"Would you tell me please which way I ought to go from here?"

"That depends a good deal on where you want to get to," said the cat.

Alice responds, "I don't much care where."

"Then it doesn't much matter which way you go!"

"As long as I get **somewhere**," Alice added as an explanation

"Oh, you're sure to do that," said the cat, "if you only walk long enough."

The metaphor I like to use is the person who consults a travel agent to make plans for a vacation. He tells the agent that he doesn't want to go to Baltimore.

"No problem. I won't send you to Baltimore. Where *do* you want to go?"

"Well, I sure don't want to go to New York. I can't afford to stay at a hotel there."

"Okay, where *do* you want to go?"

For every answer in which the person tells the agent only what he does **not** want, he is no closer to having *any* vacation, much less his desired one.

It is very important to stay positive in defining our goals rather than focusing on what you *don't* want. What you say to yourself (the internal language you use) to define our goals as a positive outcomes will determine our success in getting them. *When you make a goal clear, colorful, distinct, and passionate enough, you will achieve it.* When you visualize yourself in possession of your new eating habits, looking the way you want to look, your unconscious will adapt to it as if it were true. You are pulled into that vision as if it was real. It is important to keep this image in the forefront of our awareness, particularly in contexts or situations where food choices are involved. You must make that goal very specific in terms of the weight, or size you want to achieve and maintain:

"I want to weigh ____ pounds and wear size ____ clothes, which will fit me comfortably." You can specify the size of the clothes you will be wearing when you have reached your goal weight and imagine what they will look like when they fit you well.

Whenever you generate tangible, measurable objectives to describe goals, your internal images become real and compelling. On the other hand, if you **only** focus on what you **don't** want, you will have an *absence* of a specific, positive outcome which will attract your attention and energy. Since your brain requires an object to focus on, you will actually get **more** of what you don't want.

> *Annie:*
>
> *Annie had struggled with weight all of her life. She had been a "plump" little girl who grew into a "fat" woman. At her initial visit, with great sadness, she referred to her struggle as a "losing" battle. At the ripe old age of thirty-eight, her primary care physician told her she was a candidate for a heart attack if she did not change her eating and exercise habits. Annie considered me her "port of last resort." She had been so beaten down that when I asked her to tell me her goal weight, she could not even begin to imagine being at any other weight.*
>
> *The first step in achieving anything of importance is to set a specific goal on which to focus her attention. Together, we reviewed the criteria of establishing a well-formed outcome as it is defined above,*

and reframed this concept as "playing the game."
Annie laughed and enjoyed the humor of thinking
about resolving her problem as a "game." It was very
different for Annie to think of achieving any posi-
tive outcome, since she despised her weight and body
structure.   The last time she had been weighed, the
scale registered 215 pounds. I suggested that she set
an initial, arbitrary goal just to get started. As she
would be successful at achieving the initial goal, she
could confidently continue her journey to success. She
decided on 190 pounds. She stated that this weight
would allow her to drop down a whole dress size.
This was a big step for her. Amid the many tears that
she shed at that moment, Annie described the emo-
tion as signifying that she was "on her way."

2. Oriented to the Future

It is impossible to achieve anything different for yourself when you focus on the past. Your past represents ideas that have not worked out as successfully as you thought they would. If they had been workable, you would not be searching for alternatives. There is an old saying, "If you *conceive* it, and *believe* it, you will *achieve* it." When you structure your outcome positively and precisely into your future, you can program your mind more efficiently to notice relevant opportunities, formulate effective plans, and respond to the realities of the world so your objectives are met.

A story is told of William James, credited with the
creation of Pragmatism, as a philosophy, and the
origination of Behavioral Psychology, which provides
a helpful example. He grew up in a New England

home which used a wood stove to heat the house. It was his chore to stoke the fires in the wood stove early in the morning. It must have been a struggle to get out of a warm, quilt bed onto an icy cold floor to get his clothes on each morning. He related that while he was still in bed, he imagined already being in his warm clothes, standing by the hot stove, waiting for his mother to fix breakfast.

You have always been taught that it is 'useless to cry over spilt milk' or 'water under the bridge'; or the 'past is a cancelled check' (substitute your own favorite cliché here). You can't go back to the past, and do things over to fix any mistakes. You can only go forward in time, learn from your mistakes, and *then* do things differently.

Planning your future focuses on your objectives, dreams, and ambitions and creates hope, energy, and enthusiasm for achieving those goals, rather than wallowing in depression and despair that you haven't achieved them yet. When you look forward and put a positive plan into action, every day is a new opportunity to make your future real. You will be creating a model of your future as a reference point from which to chart your progress, and to remind you of what you are working so hard to achieve.

It is essential to focus on the possibilities of the future in order to transform your dreams into reality, rather than looking to all the failed strategies from the past. You can usually tell you are focused on the past when the image you conjure in your mind's eye reminds you of an earlier time when you were younger. An image in the future takes into account the age you will be when you have succeeded.

Annie's past had been so emotionally devastating that she was rather glad to have a reason to let go of it. To make sure her goal was future-oriented, Annie was asked to first create an image from her past. I asked her if she could remember the last time she weighed herself. Annie immediately shifted her eyes to the upper left, where she mentally stored visual memories from her past, and reported that it was about a week ago in her doctor's office. I then invited her to shift her eyes, turn her head and shoulders to the opposite direction. She focused her gaze in the direction of her future (the upper right hand quadrant of her visual field), and imagined what she wanted to look like when she was at her goal weight. When she set up that intermediate weight goal of 190 pounds in her mind, she had something important to look forward to that was different from focusing on her next meal. She acknowledged that this was a very different image than the last time she could recall being at that weight in the past.

3. Self-Initiated and Maintained

Making the changes you want must be in your own power, as opposed to depending on the actions or attitudes of anybody else. It's really hard to influence, much less control, another person's behavior. You actually have to be your own Santa Claus. When the outcomes result from your own efforts, they are not only more important to you, they also have a greater impact on influencing your future behavior effectively.

You can't rely on anyone else to achieve your weight goals and outcomes for you. No one is holding a gun to your head and insisting that you eat something fattening. Nor is anyone holding a weapon to force you to eat "slimming and healthy" foods. People close to you may be encouraging, nagging, or sometimes even discouraging. They may be inspiring to your success, or engage in sabotage to diminish your resolve. If *you* don't take the responsibility for bringing your own objectives into reality, you'll get bogged down in excuses, procrastination, disappointment, and frustration. The good news is that you also get all the credit when you succeed. The only person that can "make" you be in control of what you weigh is *you*. As the television character, Gomer Pyle was so proud of remarking, ***"Surprise! Surprise! Surprise!"***

Part of the internal determination, guts, and drive that makes any achievement possible comes about because the achievement is *worth* the effort it will take. We will be exploring the necessary hierarchy of internal values in the next chapter. From these values, you can develop a plan of action, with all the necessary steps spelled out, that feels comfortable and doable as you put it to use.

> *Annie agreed to keep a concurrent log of everything she chose to put in her mouth. She was to record the time of day, a specific description of what she ate, the quantity of food, how it was prepared (fried, broiled, steamed, etc.), any triggering activity, and her emotional state. Annie reported that this was her most challenging task; sometimes she would forget to record all the information or sometimes she would misplace the spiral notebook she used. Nevertheless, she was able to successfully record most of her eating habits with consistency and accuracy.*

Keeping a log has a three-fold purpose: the first of which is for Annie to be accountable to herself for her choices by recording them. Second, she would stay conscious of her choices; and third, she would have a concrete understanding of the habitual behavior of overeating and the behavioral triggers that accompanied these choices.

4. Behavioral in Specific Situatins

Defining behaviors and situations specifically means you will know **how** and **when** your goals are achieved. This will identify exactly what you will be *doing,* and how you will be feeling when you achieve your goals.

They help determine your plan of **behavior** whenever you're around food, whether you are at the grocery store, in a restaurant, at a party, as a guest in someone's home, or even at your own dining table? When are you most vulnerable to temptation? When do you most want the most restraint?

Everyone needs some structure in life. You get up early enough to arrive at work on time. Your credit suffers if you don't pay your bills when they are due. As a responsible person, you adopt a budget for the money you need, so you don't spend more than you take in.

Now let's think about how this is relevant to achieving your goal weight. Appropriate weight management requires the same kind of organization and persistence that you use when you set an alarm clock to get up in the morning. Winning your weight war requires prior planning, and a personal commitment. Establish a "food" budget which defines how much of the high calorie or high fat food you decide to put in your mouth. Instead of feeling restricted and deprived, you will make progress toward your goal, feel in control, and enhance your self-esteem.

> *Annie thought of her eating schedule and log as the structure that would help her be in charge of her eating habits. Being a visual person, she enjoyed having a specific, objective record of her decisions. She could compare the record of what she ate with what she read on the bathroom scale. Annie could immediately see the relationship between what she*

ate and what she weighed. She could then evaluate what she could change to get the results she wanted. Annie felt accountable and validated as she focused on the external, objective measurement. It became more of a game as she experimented with changing what she ate and noticing the effects of these different eating habits.

5. Freedom from Equivocations

A verbal equivocation is a subtle signal from our unconscious minds that indicates some concern or internal objection to achieving the proposed outcomes. You can recognize emotional equivocations in recognizing the "language of doubt". It's important to identify and honor those internal concerns or considerations to resolve inner conflicts or potential sabotages.

If you want to succeed in winning your weight war, it is important to frame these outcomes in terms that have the best chance for success. Conventional wisdom has known for a long time that anything done "half-heartedly" is only "half done". The main stumbling blocks that prevent clients from successfully achieving the goals they *say* they want are that the goals are vague, unspecified, and tentative.

If you find yourself using equivocal language and tentative words—"I'll try", "maybe", "I'll work on it", "I might", "be able to", "I guess" , "I kind of think", I'd like to" —it implies to your unconscious mind that you have doubts about your goals. Using this language may mask genuine, reality-based concerns that must be addressed, honored, and relieved before a successful outcome can be realized. Equivocations are those "escape clauses" that convince your brain that no real commitment to achieving your goal exists. Such words diminish your energy and enthusiasm to achieve any goal or outcome.

For example, **'trying'** is an invitation to failure. Think about a pen (or pencil) lying on the floor. If you want to pick it up, what do you need to do? If you pick it up immediately, you are no longer "trying," but you are actually succeeding in picking up the pen. Engage in a short experiment. If you were to 'try' to pick it up by **just** stretching out your hand as far down as it would go, you might be straining your muscles to unsuccessfully reach it. You are tempted to say, *"Look how hard I'm trying"* – and you would be absolutely right! A different approach to being successful is required.

"What would you have to do in addition to stretching out your hand?" It may mean that you have to bend further at the waist, or actually get off your seat and bend at the knees to achieve the objective. "Trying" only means that there are more steps necessary in order to succeed. If you don't know them yet and need information from others, or require additional help to carry out those steps, then you are on your way to success. A vocabulary and mindset that is positive, firm, determined and resolute is required to achieve success: *"I will, I can, and I am determined to accomplish my goal."*

When thinking of things as impossible, it may be helpful to remember that the world today is filled with such things as computers, an international space station, and even cell phones, which my grandfather's generation thought to be *impossible.*

> *Annie did not have any internal conflict, which generally makes up emotional equivocation, because she wanted to change her weight so desperately. What was more of a problem was the habitual uncertainty that she could actually succeed in obtaining her goal. Creating a sense of determination and patience for*

making progress in "baby steps" was the strategy we decided to select. Annie recalled those times when she had to be patient in accomplishing objectives successfully, and when she had remained persistent in overcoming emotional or situational "roadblocks."

Summary:

Accomplishing a goal will seem easy when it is defined in specific terms. Then that achievement becomes a forgone conclusion. Being effectively motivated requires that you know what you want, can recognize it, and be excited and enthused about the achievement.

Success is a state of mind although the specific criteria will vary depending on the values of each person. Remember that success in managing weight is an ongoing experience; an ongoing process rather than an event that ends suddenly. It has to be so important to you, that it is worth the effort that it will take to make it happen. It is vital to create a representation of a realistic outcome which will be **so** compelling that it will pull you into it. All the relevant concerns or drawbacks are taken into account to prevent remorse.

Stated in positive language which focuses your brain on what you want to achieve

Oriented to the future rather than to failed attempts from the past

Self-initiated and maintained independent of the actions of others

Behavioral and contextualized easily defined and connected to situations where the behavior is desired

Free of equivocations or "language of doubt" Change equivocal language and tentative words, such as: **"I'll try," "maybe…," "I'll**

work on it.", "I might", "I want to be able to…", "I guess I'll….", "I kinda think", "I'd like…." to definitive, positive statements which have certainty and confidence.

Resolving these internal conflicts, equivocations, or doubts is the focus of the next chapter, giving you specific strategies to change your automatic negative mindset which prevents your winning your weight struggles.

CHAPTER 3

Strategy Two: Get Rid of the "Losing" Mentality

The Three Little Kittens
– Anonymous

The three little kittens lost their mittens, and they began to cry.

"Oh, Mother dear, We sadly fear,

Our mittens we have lost."

"What? Lost your mittens?

You naughty kittens!

Then you shall have no pie.

The three little kittens found their mittens,

And they began to cry,

"Oh Mother dear, look here, look here!

Our mittens we have found!"

"Oh, found your mittens?

You good little kittens!

Then you shall have some pie."

The three little kittens put on their mittens,

And soon ate up the pie!"

"Meow! Meow! Meow!"

The following statement is probably the most important concept in this book:

*"**Words matter to your unconscious awareness, and they influence the behaviors that follow as a result!**"*

Those words that make up whatever internal dialogue you use to interpret the world determine how you feel about yourself (your self-concept) as well as any decisions that you make about your life.

Lose versus Win

Everyone experiences losses at different times in their lives, all of them considered bad! We can lose time, money, friends, games—lots of things (even our mittens!)—in addition to losing people whom we love and value. We would go to great lengths to avoid such losses if we could. Do you panic when you discover that you've lost the car keys? People feel terrible when they experience losses in the stock market. I was really upset when I realized that I had lost all my notes for a speaking presentation. Perhaps you are someone who gets distressed when losing your orientation and direction in heavy traffic. Some people get depressed for days when their favorite sports team loses a big game. In all of these situations we experience a helpless feeling because we cannot do anything to repair what happened. Losing is not very pleasant or productive. It would be very difficult to find an outcome that would be satisfying if we continue to maintain a mindset of negativity. *The* worst thing is that we really can't do anything about it. Loss is something that happens *to* us, sometimes in spite of our best efforts to avoid it.

Losing, as a concept, implies that something of value or importance is no longer available, or is being taken away from you. We have been trained from the beginning—often driven by our earliest values and memories—that we **need** to find those things we lose. It is unreasonable to make negative suggestions to the brain, and still expect positive results. We *gain* weight back because there seems to be an innate, hard-wired compulsion to get back what you have lost. This accounts for the back-and-forth yo-yo effect of crash dieting.

Passive Connotation of 'Lose'

Not only a negative word, losing is also a *passive* word. In this culture, losing implies that you have no control over being separated from something valuable. You then feel compelled to "find" those elements in your life that have been "lost." If you look up synonyms for "lose", you will find such meanings as: *defeated, go down, fail, go under, go astray, confuse, puzzle, misplace, disorient, waste, squander, exhaust, bereave,* and others that seem to be equally undesirable.

Choose Active Words

To make changes to which we are committed, we must use **strong and active verbs that have positive connotations.** Active case verbs will energize, motivate, and inspire us to move toward achieving vivid, understandable, and appealing outcomes.

An excess of anything in your homes that you no longer want, or have a need for, is usually called "junk" or "garbage." It's interesting to observe that no one ever uses the word "lose" to describe what we do with garbage. We "throw it out, get rid of it, trash it, or dump it." These are *action* words that connote taking control or doing something to change or fix what is wrong.

When we are overweight, we have an *excess* of pounds or fat that we don't want. In the same way that we don't *lose* garbage or excess elements in our lives, we often don't succeed in the struggle to "lose" weight as that implies to our unconscious minds that we want to "find" it again. Let's use such action words as: **"drop, shed, reduce, take off,**

get rid of, dispose of, or dump." These words give us the power of strength, choice, ability, entitlement, and control.

Adopt a Winning Mindset

"Win," "gain," or *"find"* are generally considered to be the polar opposite of *lose*, and have the connotation of a positive outlook, energy, and state of mind. Success in getting control over your weight, and maintaining it depends on a "winning" mindset rather than a "losing" mentality. **A winning mindset is the most positive state you can enjoy. It defines success and victory as you overcome obstacles, and draw upon your knowledge, your positive energy and motivation as well as your courage and commitment. You feel like a winner when you achieve your goals.**

We like to *find* things that we have lost, or to *find* our way back. We want to *gain* prestige, make *gains* in the stock market, gain perspective, gain friends, or gain courage as examples. We **gain** the benefits of being at our goal weight! These are all positive—and powerful! We like to *win* games, win a war, or a battle; win a bet, or win a victory over our challenges or struggles. The *winning* strategies to change our weight involve assessing all the benefits and values to be gained in achieving our goals. These benefits will range from the most trivial to the most important to us.

Focus on Positive Factors

When you focus on all the positive factors that being at your goal weight will *gain* or *win* for you, you can generate a sense of personal power, control, influence or confidence that you want to have over decisions in your life. For those who are more highly motivated to avoid what they *don't* want rather than to set a specific goal, it is important to include any possible negative outcomes as counterexamples of what would happen if they were to continue to eat in the same old ways that caused excess weight.

Annie complained that whenever she considered "going on a diet she was already in a state of grief or mourning for the foods she believed she was "losing," "missing out on" or "leaving behind." This was her biggest sabotage to all her good intentions. She looked for the short-term gratification of a taste of chocolate in her mouth rather than the long-term gratification of reaching her goals. Annie believed it was indeed a loss of a pleasure that seemed irreplaceable after having experienced an important loss such as the recent dissolution of her marriage. It was a transforming experience to redefine the importance of the longer term gratification of looking the way she wanted to look, as well feeling proud of her anticipated success.

Benefits and Values of Obtaining Your Goal Weight

One of the best ways of evaluating the benefits and values of achieving a goal is to use a technique attributed to no less a sage than Benjamin Franklin. He would have suggested that you draw a vertical straight line down the center of a sheet of paper. First, on one side, write all the advantages of reducing your weight to match a goal that you have set: "List all the advantages, from the most trivial to the most profound, that are of value to you about getting to that goal and maintaining it. For each of those advantages that you listed, ask: What is important to me about having that advantage?"

Next, on the other side of the sheet, write all the advantages of *staying at your present weight*, both trivial and profound. Be sure to include how each advantage is important to you. There is no shame in having this outcome as a goal. At least it will be a *conscious choice*, rather than a force of habit. In any case, you will be relieved of the internal conflict with which you struggle on a daily basis.

If you decide on the latter, you can just continue eating in your usual way without giving up anything, *except* all the advantages that you listed on the left hand side of your paper. You will probably use up relatively little energy. On the other hand, it will take a great deal of effort to challenge your old beliefs, change your old eating and exercise habits, and adopt new ones that support a healthy lifestyle which improves your self-esteem and well-being.

> *Allison wrote eighteen separate advantages for getting to her goal weight compared to only four in favor of keeping her weight the way it was. Her page looked something like the following:*

Advantages of getting to goal weight:

1. Knee Comfort
2. Going up and down stairs
3. Breathing easily
4. Buying fashionable clothes
5. Using normal airline seats
6. Feeling energetic
7. Being attractive to husband
8. Being admired by children
9. Having self-confidence
10. Respected by customers
11. Respected by colleagues
12. Setting a good example for kids
13. Feel pride
14. Protect against heart disease
15. Protect against diabetes
16. Lower high blood pressure
17. Feel comfortable at the gym
18. Practice what I preach about taking responsibility

Advantages of staying at present weight:

19. Enjoying food I like
20. Keep the clothes I have
21. Eating comfort foods
22. Enjoying myself at parties

What's important about these things to me?

> *Short-term pleasure; Socializing; Feeling comfort when stressed*

What's important about these things to me?

> *Integrity, Self-esteem, Taking responsibility for my health. Physical comfort when I move. Respect from others.*

Making this evaluation is perhaps the single most critical issue in building up motivation and commitment that makes all the effort you are going to put into this endeavor possible and worthwhile. When you identify your most powerful core, personal values, and match your behaviors to them, they become the **most powerful motivation** you can use to accomplish any challenge. Identifying and operating from the framework of these important values and benefits of your weight goal enables you to make decisions from the **'bottom of your heart'** or what's really important to you about being at your goal weight. These values override the habitual urges or food cravings that emotional reactions stimulate.

When asked to make this list, almost everyone puts health first, referring to it in preferential terms. The irony is that health tends to be a secondary benefit, almost the "icing on the cake" (pardon the cliché) of being at your goal weight. The highly effective motivation comes from what you can **do** for yourself when you have that health.

It is important to be honest when making these lists. Including even the most trivial benefits on those lists often allows you to discover the core values that are important to your self-esteem. The more components you can put into the equation that gives value to your projected goal, the more valuable that goal will become. This long list of benefits and values will often be a major asset in countering fears or the potential sabotages that could interfere with achieving your goal weight.

Fears of Deprivation

Deprivation of foods that have provided pleasure in the past is one of the most common fears that will sabotage the best intentions to reduce excess weight. It is *the* major drawback to "going on a diet". Comparing the accumulated value of all those positive benefits of being at your goal weight to the imagined, present value of high calorie foods, you can recognize that **the only "deprivation" you will experience is that of depriving yourself of *all* those positive benefits. Now <u>that's</u> something important to be afraid of!**

Although the following points may seem harsh, they are factors to consider, as you truthfully evaluate what's in it for you to be at your goal weight.

When you think about buying new smaller sizes in clothes, you might also consider that you are setting a good example for your children. Your children look to you to teach them how to take care of their physical health and appearance. It is hard to drive home these points when you are "out of control" as far as your eating habits are concerned. Personal pride, as well as professional respect from your colleagues is very much at stake when you consider that wearing clothes that are loose in order to hide your expanding waistline may not give you the professional appearance that you want. First impressions being what they are, it may be hard to shake negative assumptions about professional skills based on appearances. Like it or not, people on the job do tend to evaluate competence based on appearance (hence the conventional wisdom that 'first impressions are important'). To overcome these negative "first impressions", you often have to work harder to gain professional respect than your more slender colleagues. Allison Van Dusen contributed an article entitled 'Is Your Weight Affecting Your Career?' in ***Forbes.Com*** in May of 2008 which confirms concerns that "*…weight based discrimination affects every aspect of employment from hiring to firing, promotions, pay allocation, career counseling and discipline….*" It's not just in your imagination.

Resolve Inner Conflicts

Internal conflicts or wanting an outcome on one hand, but having concerns or even small objections which interfere with successfully achieving victory. It takes discovering an inner peace to resolve this kind of conflict. As an example of how this works, consider Barbara's story.

Barbara:

Barbara, a 38-year-old homemaker, had allowed her weight to balloon out to nearly 200 pounds. She said that she thought her marriage was strong, but her husband had begun to comment about his concerns that she was putting her health in danger by carrying too much weight. He would "joke" that their "mattress was in danger of collapse." Barbara recognized that she had an intense internal conflict about even the thought of weighing what she said she wanted. It would need to be put to rest before she could fully commit to doing what was required to achieve success. We first identified the elements of the conflict, both parts of which were equally relevant, and equally valuable in her life.

Barbara realized that the conflict originated with the fact that the majority of her friends were also overweight, but didn't seem to care. It was like a band of "sisters" who were emotionally supportive of each other. The downside was that they seemed to take great delight in disparaging the efforts of several people to "go on a diet." The restaurants they frequented had very few "healthy" selections. Barbara valued their friendships, and believed she would be considered a "traitor" by this circle of friends if she reduced her weight.

I asked Barbara to create two different images to represent the two opposing sides, one in each hand. The first was to imagine wearing a "kicky", clingy red dress, feeling really special as an image in her right hand. The left hand held onto her need for friendship as Barbara imagined her good friends smiling at her in approval. She closed her eyes as she alternated her awareness to focus intensely on the positive intentions and important needs of each position. The question she posed to **each** side of her conflict was, **"As a part of me, what are you attempting to get for me, or do for me that is important in my life?"**

The "Slender Self" (represented by the red dress) wanted to be healthy, sexually attractive to her husband, proud of herself, and respected at her office so she could advance to an upper management position.

The "Circle of Friends" image wanted to keep the connection and support of her friends. She had developed a taste for the pizzas, pastas, and sweet treats they had been sharing. Barbara didn't want to sacrifice the good company she was enjoying.

Next, Barbara asked herself what were the significant, positive values that inspired these positive intentions for each side, so that the "opposing" parts could truly appreciate the advantages, purposes, and importance that were so important that both sides could agree to work together to ensure the realization *of these values for the good of the whole person. Any alternative behaviors which could satisfy those opposite intentions would have to respect all of the values that had been identified, rather than being stuck in the bind of an either/or position.*

It was as if these two parts of her were meeting as equals for the first time.

The values that were true of both sides were **loyalty, flexibility, optimism, and respect.** *Barbara recognized that if she were loyal to herself in respecting her health needs, as well as preserving the health of her marriage, she could preserve her self-respect, and count on her friends to accept her healthy decisions, if they were really her friends. She could be in charge of ordering very healthy lunches without a specific explanation, and could suggest other restaurants which had more varied menus. She could join them for social activities, and order what she needed to stay loyal to her commitment. If her friends could not accept her decision, she was comfortable to either ignore the trivial, snide comments, or to just cultivate other circles of friends. As Barbara allowed these factions to grant mutual respect and honor to each other, Barbara's two hands slowly moved toward each other until they joined together: as if both parts of this conflict were finally working together to resolve any value differences and to achieve a unified outcome. Barbara reported that she finally felt at peace inside herself.*

Self-respect

Most people who are highly motivated to be at their goal weight not only want to have respect from others, whether colleagues, customers, clients, or friends, but also want self-respect. If being active and energized in order to keep up with your children (or grandchildren) is important to you, it might be difficult to run up and down stairs when you are carrying twenty or thirty pounds of extra weight without getting winded, much less running around the yard to catch a deep pass or a fast lay-up at the driveway hoop.

Bob

Bob was a manager-in-training for a health management organization with aspirations for advancement. He reported that he wanted to "run pass plays" with his two sons in the yard for more than five minutes at a time, to go hiking and enjoy the outdoors the way he used to, and to sit comfortably on the seat of his bicycle. He wanted to serve as an example for his sons so they would respect him and perhaps "have me available to play with them while they are young enough to enjoy it. They might also see that if I can make changes, they can too. When Bob saw his stomach spilling over his slacks, he decided that he wanted to have the pride in his appearance that he used to have when he was in high school and college. He added that he thought his wife would be more physically attracted to him when he reduced his weight.

Bob admitted that respect from his co-workers was also important as he observed that trim and fit colleagues were often treated more seriously, and with more deference, even though they were less experienced than he was. He added several trivial benefits such as buying new clothes in Brooks Brothers (his favorite store), and wearing a thirty-six-inch belt rather than a forty-two-inch belt. The benefit that meant the most to him was the personal integrity that he would have when his personal health choices matched the values that he preached to those people who were participants in the HMO.

Bob's example is very common in terms of how people think that their weight impacts their lives. These impacts often become the driving force to help people make changes in their weight, appearance and self-image.

Annie focused on the benefits of shopping in "normal" stores and fitting into the style of clothes she enjoyed seeing in the magazines. She wanted to avoid disgusted expressions on the faces of fellow airline passengers when the flight attendant had to bring her a seatbelt extender. She wanted to go up and down steps easily and comfortably. Annie was committed to protecting her knees and ankles, which had begun to hurt when she walked. Since her family history included heart disease, Annie decided to decrease her cholesterol and fat intake so she could have a clear conscience that she was doing everything she could to protect herself. Most importantly, Annie wanted to feel pride when she looked at herself in the mirror.

When we are focused on the positive benefits of setting goals and working towards achieving them, they override the imagined, negative impacts on our lives. When there is so much at stake, it is easier to motivate ourselves to make the "right" decisions to honor our highest values.

Remind Yourself of the Benefits

Write down each one of the benefits of being at your goal weight on separate filing cards. Place one of them on your refrigerator, pantry, car, wallet, or bathroom mirror - anywhere that you would be thinking of how you look, or when you might be tempted to eat fattening foods. You can remind yourself of what is at stake. Change the cards around often, so they stay fresh and new to your eyes and to your mind.

Summary:

Get Rid of the Losing Mentality

Words matter to our unconscious awareness! Losing implies that something of value or importance is no longer available or is being taken away from us, which creates an anxiety to get that something back. We want to get rid of the passive mentality that will "weigh" us down with impotence. Any time there is an excess of material that we no longer want, have need for, or have too much of, we usually call this "garbage." The language we use is a powerful monitor of the metaphors that define our lives. We never think of "losing" garbage, but of dropping, getting rid of or shedding evidence of this excess. We can learn to generate a sense of personal power, control, energy, or desire that we want to have over the kinds of food and how much food we allow to be in our bodies in order to remain in control of our weights. It is important to make it worth our while to invest this time, energy, and in some cases, money, to achieve the goals that validate or increase our core values. When we build up the motivation and commitment that makes all the effort we are going to put into this endeavor possible and worthwhile, we access powerful, core personal values and put them to action to influence our behavior. We reduce any internal conflict that might sabotage our best efforts.

People perceive that their weight impacts their life. It is important to develop a visual model of what you want that is unique to you. This image in your mind's eye that represents you at the weight and size you want to be and creates a very powerful ally to make you successful. Chapter Four will explore this very concept in detail.

CHAPTER 4

Strategy Three: Create Your Personal Cheerleader

There are many elements in any personal environment that can be discouraging. Life can be filled with pressures, aggravations, and hassles from parents, supervisors, coworkers, children, spouses, creditors—and the list goes on. It is common to focus on these problems, rather than on those times when we feel loved, appreciated, and satisfied. When we consider the time spent and the energy invested in the struggle to reach the outcome that is wanted, it's easy to believe we are battling the eating temptations all by ourselves. It is very important to gather a support system that can energize and stoke the motivational fires before they burn themselves out.

Developing your 'cheerleading squad'

If you can share your weight goals, fears and concerns with those **who care** about you, you can ask them to help support and encourage you in all the ways that you would find the most helpful. Ironically, it often happens that no matter how much they know you and love you, they don't read your mind and have no clue about how to be helpful. You might want some people to be "gatekeepers" to keep you free of "sweet temptations". You might ask others to take the role of "warm comforters" who would be encouraging and loving in reminding you of how much getting to your goals means to you. The most important thing is to specify how you want others in your life to be helpful and supportive to you.

One thing that **no one** wants is to be teased, taunted, or abused about the efforts they are taking to make positive changes. If there are people around you who refuse to be supportive or enthusiastic about helping you achieve your goals, you may need to find your support system elsewhere. "Weight Watchers", "Jenny Craig", "Nutri-System", local hospital wellness centers or even select fitness centers can provide this kind of encouragement and support, as well as valuable information on nutrition and exercise. The people that you meet who are fellow veterans of the weight wars provide a mutual assistance and support system to validate what you are doing successfully, and to share new strategies that may work even better. They are equally open to hearing your hopes, fears, and struggles. You will be able to offer them similar kinds of support, comfort and validation, so it's a win-win situation for everyone.

When push comes to shove, you are generally on your own at the most important choice points in your day: when you shop for food, prepare it, or decide which foods to put in your mouth – as well as how much of those foods to eat. It would be nice to have your own squad of cheerleaders available to you, much the same way as all the schools have "pep squads" or the professional football teams use attractive, athletic cheerleaders to stir up the crowds. They certainly cheer when the team is ahead, but they cheer even louder with encouragement when the team is behind to "rally" the spirit of the team to use extra effort. Everyone needs a personal advocate, coach, or cheerleader to be enthusiastic and offer inspiration to keep you going when the "going gets tough". He or she knows just what to say to keep your spirits up and you can trust him or her to give you good information and advice.

A 'future-self' ally and cheerleader

What better way to make sure your "cheerleader" is completely available to you, than to create your own personal coach inside of you who will act as an advisor who could encourage you to act in your own best interest? Keeping you oriented to your future, and focused on doing what it takes to achieve the benefits of winning victory in your weight battles is best directed by an advisor who knows you better than anyone else in the world and who has a vested interest in making sure you are successful. That is your future-self, whose **very existence** is completely dependent on every decision that you make about food and exercise from this minute on, for the rest of your life.

This future-self knows more about who you are, what is important to you as well as those temptations which confront you than any other person in the world. The main advantage is that your future self is **already** at your goal weight, and has been successful at achieving the many small victories necessary to win the war. She has a very different perspective about the important choices that are necessary to make winning possible. Use this future self as an effective filter to overcome your old eating and snacking habits and replace them with appropriate, healthy choices in the kinds of food as well as the quantity that you consume.

After understanding the rationale for creating an internal cheerleader and ally, the first step is to make an image in your minds eye that represents you being at your goal weight. In addition to having a vivid, clear model of what you want to look like, and how you want others to see you, you will have an objective to work towards that clearly reminds you of all the benefits that symbolize and embody your values, and which you identified as being important.

Diane

A fifty-five years young grandmother, Diane made herself available on a daily basis to care for her grandchildren while her daughter worked. She wanted to get back in shape so she could keep up with the physi-

cal demands of childcare. When it was suggested that she would find an internal ally useful, Diane was very intrigued. She closed her eyes, and thought of what she wanted to look like at her goal weight. Diane mentioned, in passing, that the she was thinking of a photograph of herself, twenty years ago; which was the last time she had weighed what she wanted.

The following is a transcript of our session to create her "future self ally":

"How do you feel when you look at that image, Diane? What meaning does it have for you?"

Diane: "Well, it looks good, but I guess it seems very far off. I don't feel very excited about it."

"That's not surprising since it's a picture of you from your past. It represents all the attempts you made in the past which were unsuccessful. You want an image which is age appropriate, and created as a goal yet to be achieved. (This is true even if you have been at your goal weight previously.) In your imagination, make sure you see that image from head to toe, paying special attention to the facial expressions. Now, one at a time, make sure that image is:

- life-sized
- three dimensional
- clearly focused
- in vivid color
- a movie
- Free of a particular situation or context, so it is available to you at any time you want it.

(Pause) How far away is that image?"

When Diane reported that this image was some distance from her across the room, I invited her to move it close enough to talk to on an intimate basis (within five feet) – and add a sound track.

Diane: *"I can see it much more clearly now. My hair is still salt and pepper gray, but it looks very inviting."*

"That is your future self. To bring her into your reality, she is completely dependent <u>for her very existence</u> on all the decisions that you make about what kinds of food you will put in your mouth as well as determining how much of that food to eat from this moment on for the rest of your life. Think about how often physical exercise will be part of your life. Make that image as vivid and real as you can, and if it is important enough for you to want it in your future, it will <u>pull</u> you into it.

Now, I invite you to mentally step inside that future self, and imagine what you will feel, think and see as you move around inside that body, weighing what she weighs, and looking at the world through her eyes. Pay particular attention to how she evaluates her food choices and how much she wants to eat."

(About 30 seconds later)

"Now shift back into your present self, and tell me how that was."

Diane: "Wow! Whooh! I felt so light! I was moving so easily and painlessly. She seemed so proud of picking foods that had very little fat, even when people offered her chocolate desserts. If that happens I am more and more confident about succeeding. It's exciting to imagine that I can do that!"

"Spend a moment of time inside, now, just enjoying the possibility of that future. (Pause) Now, I would invite you to make a <u>commitment</u> to that future self in your own words, from the very "bottom of your heart" to do whatever it takes to bring her into reality. It is between you and what you imagine that you will look like when you reach your goal weight. This commitment must be taken very seriously by you, because it is made at the level of your highest values, based on what is <u>genuinely</u> important to you. It becomes almost a "covenant" for you with that future self. Notice the response. (Pause) Take as long as you need, and let me know when that commitment is made."

Diane: (After about two minutes) "Okay, I did it."

"What was her response to your commitment?"

Diane: "She was pretty skeptical at first, but I kept on insisting that this time, I was taking myself seriously. Finally, she said she was really glad."

"Ask her for her help as your ally in helping you make all the wise decisions about the food you eat. The fact is that she has already succeeded in ac-

complishing that goal. She can remind you of all of those important benefits that you identified that were important about getting to that weight, and maintaining it. Will she agree to that role?"

Diane: "Oh my, yes! She actually seems enthusiastic."

"Great! Now, I would like you to see her in your future as a guide and a coach to help you make choices about what you put into your mouth to eat. Let's experiment with this a little. Put an image of your favorite dessert (say cheesecake) in one hand, and that image of your future self, in the other. Which seems more appetizing to you? Which one would you go for?"

Diane: "It's no contest. My future self runs away with that decision."

"Now think of those French fries that you loved to eat and compare eating them with having the benefits of that future self."

Diane: "They don't even look appetizing anymore! That's amazing! I didn't think I could ever feel that way. It reminds me of the time I quit smoking. At the time, I had to continue to say to myself: 'No I won't do that to myself. It's not worth it.' I hear that same expression as I look at those foods."

"This is the key to making positive choices. Keep that future self in front of you. Remember that nothing goes into your mouth without making that com-

parison. Use all the resolve and determination that goes along with that image to be all the encouragement that you need to make that image real. (Pause.) Now, take a moment of time to determine if you are feeling deprived in any way after making those decisions."

Diane: "Surprisingly, no. I am really encouraged and excited about keeping my commitment and getting to my goal. Go figure!"

Diane's response is typical of most people. This strategy is *very* popular, mainly because it is useful in so many contexts. Whether you practice making those choices in your mind's eye, or are making those healthy decisions in real time, before you decide what or how much to put in your mouth, you can feel in control.

Keep a Journal

It is important to have a written record of what you put into your mouth. It's easy to forget what we eat one day to another, particularly since we often take food and our consumption of it for granted. Clients have told me that they didn't understand how they could have put on weight when they really "hadn't changed their eating habits". Once they started keeping a food journal, recording the day, time, choices, quantity, and emotional mood at the time they started to eat, they were floored to discover just how many calories they consumed. The connection of emotion to eating was painfully obvious. They began to appreciate the objective perspective that the journal provided. Diane was very happy to have a way of keeping track of her progress. *"Every day that I could actually see a difference, I could be very proud of myself, even though I hated the task at first."*

Another option is to include all the exercise that you do each day whether it's incidental such as vacuuming; or very purposeful such as running or working out. It's also an opportunity to focus on how the day's events have impacted your emotions whether producing nervousness, sadness, excitement, or anger. It's possible to trace how these emotions trigger your eating habits.

Memory Mantras

One effective way to reinforce your commitment to yourself is to find a "mantra" (or two) to repeat, reminding you of your power to make appropriate decisions. Feel free to use any of the suggestions below, or create your own.

> **"Shed the dread!**
> **Shed the Bread!**
> **Shed the Spread!"**
> **"The essence of "Waste" is to eat more of high calorie foods, when what you want, is to weigh less."**
> **"Don't let food go to "waste" on your waist"!**
> **"A moment on the lips; forever on the hips"**
> **"Nothing tastes as good as being slender feels!"**

Write down **your** favorite sayings! Repeat them often, understanding the meaning of what you are saying to yourself; then act appropriately on each saying.

Summary:

It is very important to affiliate with positive people in support systems that provide encouragement, empathy and understanding of the struggle you are going through. Families and friends are the first line of support. If for any reason, they are unwilling or incapable of giving you this kind of positive energy, seek out those commercial groups who have specialized training, knowledge, and experience in helping clients get to their weight goals.

In addition, you need an ***internal*** **ally** or cheerleader to help you make decisions, in real life situations, or when no one else is around. This constructed representation of your desired outcome in your future serves as a vivid, visual reference for all the benefits of achieving your goal.

1. Construct a vivid, internal, visual, three-dimensional image of what you would like to look like and doing all the things you want to do when you have attained your goal.

2. Check to make sure it is indeed a future representation, rather than one from your past.

3. Make it life-size, three dimensional, clearly focused, in vivid color, a movie, no more than five feet away with no particular context.

4. Add a sound track.

5. When it is just the way you want it, step inside of it and feel what it feels like to live inside that skin of your personal future self.

6. Make a commitment to that future self to do whatever it takes to bring her into reality.

7. Ask for her help as your ally.

8. Use this future self as a guide and coach to encourage you in making food choices.

Keep a food journal to track eating, exercising and emotions. Find an easily remembered saying or **mantra** to remind you of your mission!

The next chapter will introduce you to strategies of setting limits and boundaries on the quantity of food that you eat. How do you know when to start eating, and how to generate a stop signal when you are comfortable rather than waiting until you feel full?

CHAPTER 5

Strategy Four: Internal 'Signal Corps' A Fistfull of Food Will Fill You!

Sensory Awareness

How do you know when you are hungry? What physical sensations do you experience when you are hungry? These are not abstract questions – but very practical ones as you focus on the specific struggles to win your most personal war. Most people with weight problems eat even though they are not particularly hungry. Consider that the concept of "hunger" that middle class Americans experience is more of a *psychological* awareness than a physical one. For example, if you have been sitting at your desk for a long time, you might feel groggy, bored, or even overwhelmed. It may be easy to attribute that internal feeling with needing or wanting something to eat, when in fact getting up, stretching, moving around or just focusing on a new task would be the invigoration that is needed. It's common for psychological hunger to be tied to the clock, which determines the degree of hunger you experience—as in, "It's time to eat!" Many people confuse hunger with thirst. It might be even be mingled with the desire to be connected socially or professionally, *"I go along with the group when they go out to lunch – even after I ate the midday snack I brought with me."*

It is not easy to develop a sensory awareness for those internal cues which can differentiate the subtle difference between being hungry and feeling comfortable. Becoming sensitized to your own internal sensations that you define as physical 'hunger' requires a great deal of conscious thought. You can have a means of evaluating your progress toward feeling comfortable rather than waiting until you are full. You will be more in control of knowing when to start eating, how much to eat, and when to stop.

Location and size of your stomach

It is important to understand where your stomach is located. When asked to describe the exact location of the stomach in their body, many people will put their hands on the lower abdomen. Nope! That is where women have their reproductive organs. Men actually have more room for intestines – both large and small. It's no wonder women who have had children have to work **harder** to get a flat abdomen. The uterus is stretched with help from every child.

Actually, if you put your finger at your solar plexus where your rib cage comes together, your stomach is slightly under that on your left side between the esophagus and your intestines. It is a muscular, elastic, gourd-shaped organ which changes its shape and size depending on whether you are sitting, standing or lying down, as well as the amount of food inside. It is no wonder that the sensation of stomach acid seeping back into the lower esophagus is referred to by the expression, "heartburn." Your stomach is an organ, and will adjust and stretch to contain any amount of food you put into it. If you eat until you are full, you will continue to gain weight.

The reason that physicians perform bariatric or gastric by-pass surgery is to artificially reduce the size of your stomach. **Your natural stomach is only a little larger than the size of your fist.** Make a fist with one hand. That is a visual representation of the size of your stomach relative to the size of your body frame and bone structure. This means that if you only eat the volume of **"a fist-full of food"**, you will be comfortable rather than stuffed. When you wait until you have new sensations of physical hunger before you eat again, you will be in control of your weight. This is not to say you can get to your goals by eating "fistfuls" of sweets or carbohydrates. A balanced selection of protein, vegetables, and complex carbohydrates will guarantee nourishment while your stomach retains its normal elasticity and size. You can efficiently use the calories that you consume for the nourishment of your body. When you create an objective image, description, or mindset such as a "fist-full of food" which can measure how you define being 'comfortable' in your stomach, you will never stuff yourselves into obesity. This may mean you may get "hungry" more often, but as long as you only eat small portions no larger than the size of your fist, you will be in control of your weight.

Criteria of Hunger

Let's create some meaningful criteria of hunger that are sensory based so that you know inside when to start eating – as well as when to stop. Hunger is a sensation of deprivation marked by a dull pain, discomfort, or intense stomach contractions sometimes accompanied by feelings of weakness. It can be distinguished from an appetite by the degree of intensity associated with hunger and the pleasure experienced when anticipating food.

The following chart offers a visual representation of how to tell when to eat, and even more importantly, when to stop eating. The real trick is to stop eating when you feel **comfortable,** rather than waiting until you feel full. Being full stretches your stomach. A vicious circle follows as you have to **keep** eating more and more to feel as full as you did before.

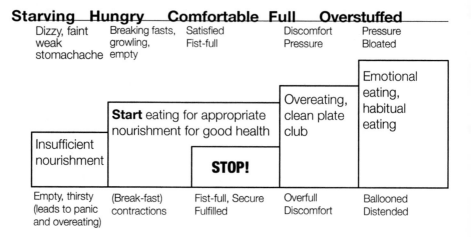

Starving	Hungry	Comfortable	Full	Overstuffed
Dizzy, faint weak stomachache	Breaking fasts, growling, empty	Satisfied Fist-full	Discomfort Pressure	Pressure Bloated

Insufficient nourishment

Start eating for appropriate nourishment for good health

Overeating, clean plate club

Emotional eating, habitual eating

STOP!

Empty, thirsty (leads to panic and overeating)	(Break-fast) contractions	Fist-full, Secure Fulfilled	Overfull Discomfort	Ballooned Distended

A "Fistfull" of Food

Portion control is your most important consideration. The measure which deserves your attention is the size of your fist. If you limit the amount of food you eat to no more than the size of your fist, you will have much more control over what you weigh. When your stomach stretches larger than the size of your fist, you will consistently have the sensations of "needing more food" to believe that you are satisfied.

Your overweight body does not metabolize food as efficiently as that of your more slender friends. Winning your personal weight battle does not mean you will "never" eat things you like. It means that you constantly evaluate how important it is to you to weigh what you want, and compare this to how important it is for you to eat a particular food. It does mean adopting a lifestyle shift in which you remain **conscious** of your food decisions, for the rest of your life.

Eating large amounts of sugars and fats will detract you from winning your weight war. This chart focuses on recognizing the sensations of being normally hungry such as in the morning after a 12 hour fast. (It's not accidental that we call the first meal of the day "breakfast".) Stay inside the "fistfull of food" concept and you will develop an accurate physical sensation of what "comfort" feels like. Eat slowly enough to stay conscious of the gradation of those physical sensations – and define **that** as satisfaction, You can stop eating at that point and feel secure, knowing you have taken good care of yourself.

Carol:

*In response to a question about how long she had been battling her weight, Carol, who was a thirty-seven year-old corporate executive, recalled that she had been very thin as a little girl. When she was about seven years old, a great aunt held up her thin wrist and proclaimed in authoritative and somber tones, that "You are **so-o-o** thin, you will die of starvation!"*

That scared her so badly, that even though she would get uncomfortable, she started eating lots and lots of food to make sure she wouldn't "die of starvation."

Unfortunately, that aunt did not install a signal for Carol to stop eating. She generated only an unending need to eat, supposedly for "preservation." When I pointed out that she had no stop signal for herself, Carol began to cry, as the waste of all her efforts began to sink in.

Carol decided to create an internal sensation that she would recognize as her signal to stop eating. While Carol was relaxed, feeling secure and competent, she remembered a time when she was aware of having eaten too much. The first internal, physical cue that she identified, with some degree of embarrassment, was a feeling of heaviness and drooping in the buttocks. It was not anything that anyone else could see or identify, but Carol intuitively knew it was right for her. She thought about other times when she had experienced a similar "droopiness," but had not identified it as connected with the amount of food that she consumed. Whenever she became aware of the heaviness in her rear end, she would put her fork or spoon down, and stop eating. Carol reported continued success as she regularly used her new "comfort barometer" as she referred to it.

The main problem that sinks many a commitment is the inability to differentiate between physical hunger and emotional hunger. Because each hunger is driven by different deficiencies, each one will require a different approach to ensure satisfaction.

The emotional responses we experience in response to both positive events such as celebrations, or for negative ones, such as anger, grief or fear, are often interpreted as sensations of "hunger." Many people have been programmed from a very early age to "feed" hungers, so they eat food instead of looking for more appropriate ways to deal with the emotional issues that seem to haunt them.

Depending on past experiences and expectations, emotional hungers develop in response to real or imagined deprivations, which you sense at the depth of your being rather than in the center of your stomach. The circumstances which provoke these intense needs originate from perceptions of insult, loss, abuse, or distress. Food simply does not adequately address negative emotions of disappointment, neglect, hurt, loneliness or grief. The solutions are neither simple nor easy. They may require you to emotionally comfort that small child inside of you, who is longing to hear words of love, attention and acceptance from the only person in the world capable of giving those wonderful resources to your younger self – that is **YOU!**

Emotional hungers

Emotional hungers cry out for recognition and validation to satisfy those needs that generate your overeating; and require you to understand how you are being deprived of these important satisfactions. Finding the **internal** resources that will satisfy those needs will actually be appropriate antidotes to those emotional deficits. You need to discriminate between these different hungers so you can create more efficient and effective ways to satisfy those emotional hungers that have nothing to do with food. In fact, food is the least effective way of feeling better when you are in pain emotionally. It will only serve to produce overweight as you continue to eat more and more with less and less success at feeling better in the long term.

Another effective exercise is to replace your perception of helplessness and discouragement with a remembered experience anytime in your life when you felt determination, confidence, and energy.

Resources of Confidence and Competence

"Recall a time and place where you felt competent, confident and determined. Close your eyes, and transport yourself back through time and space to see what you see, hear what you hear (any words or sounds in that environment), notice what you say to yourself at that moment in time, and pay attention to where in your body you have those good feelings."

Annie really was energized by this exercise. She recalled her triumph when she graduated from high school as the valedictorian and received a full scholarship to college. Although the courses were challenging, she worked hard and consistently as she knew her parents would not be able to afford to pay for college. One of the clearest memories was spending her free hours in the library, missing out on social opportunities when some of her friends were "hanging out" at the coffee shop. As Annie visualized giving her valedictorian address, she was seeing the experience through her own eyes so there was movement. It was in vivid color, three-dimensional, panoramic, as well as being brightly lit and highly focused. The sounds of the auditorium were resounding in her ears, while a small part of her was cheering, **"Yay! You did it! Isn't this cool?"** Annie could feel the huge smile on her face from one ear to the other as the scene became more and more realistic. She reported the experience of being warm all over, and she was aware of her heart beating faster with the excitement.

When Annie was asked to imagine being at her goal weight, she reported that she could see herself in a bathing suit at the beach as she observed other people looking at her with smiles on their faces. She described the scene as being a little hazy with muted colors. In comparing the two, she remarked that the goal weight scene was good while the valedictorian scene had been "terrific." When I suggested that she change the focus and the colors of the second scene to make them more like the first one, she began to smile broadly. **"I think I've got it!"**

Thirst

Thirst is a deficit that is often confused with hunger. Water is not only nourishing and cleansing, but it works very well to fill you without adding calories. If you need something with a taste, add some lemon or lime wedges. Seltzer water comes in all kinds of flavors with nary a calorie in sight. Skim milk will give you the calcium you need with few fat calories. Iced tea with some lemon or iced coffee is a wonderful summertime treat. Be creative, and make a game of discovering new low calorie drink "recipes."

> *Diane was delightfully surprised when she discovered she could quench a thirst instead of eating food. Drinking seltzer water with a slice of lemon felt refreshing compared to her past habit of snacking on something hard, crunchy and often salty. She laughed when she realized eating those things actually gave her an excuse to drink something.* ***"It's like cutting out the 'middle man.'"***

Satisfy Your Taste Center

If you cringe at the thought of missing the wonderful tastes of different foods when you commit to being on a "diet," you are in good company. It is this idea that most commonly leads us to sabotage our commitment to getting to our weight goals. There are several points that can alleviate these fears.

The irony is that winning the war on your weight is **not** about 'never' having really tasty things. It is **entirely** about being discreet, practical and even discriminating. You all engage in activities with family and friends that are joyous, social, and involve food. It is foolhardy to believe that you should or could be a perpetual martyr to the cause of being slender. The concept that I like to promote is **"five steps toward your goal, one step backwards."** The backward steps are the treats that make life worthwhile. You can give yourself permission to enjoy such treats with **no guilt attached to them!** What you are monitoring is the **frequency and quantity** of those treats. Sometimes, when you have something to look forward to, it makes it much more tolerable to 'bite the bullet' for a specific time in eating sensible, nutritional foods. I like to use the metaphor of a financial budget as a similar concept. Unless you are in the same economic class as Bill Gates, most of us cannot afford to buy everything you want. Everyone has to make choices. Instead of three dressy outfits, you might need to choose which **one** that you **really** want. This decision may depend on factors such as where and how often you might wear it, color, style, how it fits, if it feels good to wear, looks nice, and finally, if it is **worth** the money you are spending. You might decide on an outfit which is made with such quality and style that it is worth paying a greater amount of money. It is realistic and practical to understand you can't do that often, or you will not have enough money for other clothes. It may be necessary to delay or refuse to buy other items of clothing to make sure your budget is kept in line. It's all about choices!

Making Choices

You can use the same reasoning to evaluate the quality and the quantity of any high calorie foods you decide to eat. You make these choices within the framework of your ultimate goals. The criteria are different in that you evaluate these choices based on how infrequently you might get to enjoy these high calorie foods. You might decide that it is important to enjoy a small quantity of some high calorie food or drink once a week. Another option is to "save up" your calories" so that, perhaps once a month, you can enjoy the many calories of a really rich dessert such as tiramisu, chocolate cake, or a dinner time treat like one of your mom's 'cheddar cheese, twice-baked potatoes".

Make sure that any particular food is **exactly** what you want at this time. Can you postpone that choice so it is not responding to "necessity" of a craving, but rather a reasoned choice? If you eat this **now**, what does it mean in terms of the quality of your life? Looking ahead, will you be pleased or upset with this choice? Instead of feeling guilty after eating high fat and high calorie foods, you can put the potential negative aftermath into your consciousness ahead of time.

Think about what healthy, low calorie foods you can consume which will offset or compensate for this enticing, delectable 'treat'. The higher in calories a food is, the less frequently you will want to consume the food in order to stay in control. Every treat should be so special, that it's "worth every calorie." I like to refer to that quality of pleasure and satisfaction that you receive from a treat as an "oral orgasm". After enjoying the treat, you can be highly motivated to get back on track with your commitment.

Gourmet vs. Glutton

A "gourmet" is one who eats selectively with a refined taste for food. A glutton eats or drinks an excess of everything that is available. To be in control of your weight, you have to be discriminating in both your choice of foods, and to be very picky about how much of that wonderful food that you eat. This will enable you to thoroughly enjoy whatever you choose to eat with enhanced satisfaction. Eating "mindfully", in which you pay particular attention to the smells, flavors, tastes and texture of food, can be almost a spiritual experience – if you take your time and stay in a state of self-conscious awareness. I call this eating everything with **relish** (the emotional kind). Your level of taste satisfaction will increase substantially.

Next time you are at your favorite restaurant waiting for your meal to arrive, do a little people watching. Notice how other diners are eating. Are they taking the time to eat slowly, and actually **taste** the food they eat? Are they eating very quickly, as if the meal was an ordeal to get through as fast as possible? If a buffet is available, how much food do they put on their plate? Are people going back for seconds or thirds?

Sensory Discrimination in the Mouth

Were you aware that your mouth is **the** most discriminating sensory organ of your body? It helps your brain differentiate between sweet, sour, bitter, salty and all the nuances in between. You can detect hints of garlic, oregano, or curry – or know when there is too much of it in your food. Think of the last meal that you considered memorable. If you closed your eyes, could you mentally imagine what it tasted like or almost smell the aroma? Can you make a picture of the surroundings that helped make that dish so memorable? I'll wager "dollars to donuts" that you relaxed, ate slowly, and thoroughly enjoyed the company or the environment.

The Rate of Eating

How fast or how slowly you eat is a definitive factor in winning your weight war. It is not accidental that your mouth is closer to your brain than it is to your stomach. You have the time and opportunity to actually evaluate your food for freshness and quality.

If our cavemen ancestors discovered that the food was spoiled, or tasted badly, they could spit it out. You have to eat slowly enough for your taste buds to detect any disgust, and spit it out. Your tongue is able to discriminate between salty, bitter, sweet and sour tastes, and working with your sense of smell, can detect the flavors of foods and the additional zest that herbs, spice seasonings offer. If you eat quickly, you will not truly appreciate the wonderful taste sensations that give you eating satisfaction. It is only when you eat slowly that you will be able to notice when you are feeling comfortable. Eating fast ensures that the cues to **stop** eating are only noticeable when you are already full, or even uncomfortably so.

There are **four major advantages to eating very slowly.**

1. Even if you have only a short time to eat, **eating slowly increases your level of satisfaction**. One forkful of food, eaten slowly and with awareness, represents the satisfaction and value of three or four forkfuls that have been consumed rapidly. You are eating less—and enjoying it more! Your mouth contains your body's most powerful taste center. The taste buds in your tongue, aided by saliva, are stimulated by each tiny bit of food. Focus your attention completely on the food you are eating. Use all of your senses. Notice the color and texture of your food. Inhale deeply to absorb and appreciate the aroma of the food you are about to eat. Take a very small portion of food on your spoon or fork. Let your lips gently pull the food off. Just allow it to stay in your mouth for a couple seconds. Let the saliva permeate the morsel of food. Begin to chew your food thoughtfully, slowly, and thoroughly before swallowing to allow all the flavors in the food to be released.

2. Eating slowly and chewing thoroughly will aid in the digestion process, as the stomach acids don't have to work so hard at producing enough acid to break down the foods.

3. You are giving your stomach a chance to adapt itself to food. Have you ever noticed that when dining in a fine restaurant that serves several courses, or even when the service is slow, you no longer feel hungry before the main course arrives? You can think of this as an opportunity that forces you to eat more slowly.

4. Eating slowly allows you to be much more conscious of controlling your portion size and to notice specifically when you have eaten enough food to be comfortable. Eating portions no larger than the size of your fist will help you reduce the size of your stomach to one that is consistent with your bone structure, height and physique. You will be eating comparably to someone who weighs what you want to weigh.

   Allison related a recent experience at a restaurant where the salad was already on the table. After those plates were cleared, the soup was brought out. The group she was with was laughing and talking, and no one realized how much time had passed before the main entrée was served. Much to her surprise, Allison felt very comfortable after having eaten the soup and salad. She asked that the entrée be placed in a "to-go" container – and thoroughly enjoyed it the following evening. The lesson she learned was that when she could take her time eating, she ate less and enjoyed it more.

Some people are tempted when the restaurant server brings the bread basket to the table.

Evelyn:

*Evelyn described the situation as being as if there were two parts of her. The conscious, responsible part inside had made up its "competent" mind to send back the bread basket so she could more thoroughly enjoy the delicious dinner she was planning to order. She had her hand out to motion "No! Stop! Take it away!" Suddenly it was as if that responsible part "went to sleep" as the server drew closer. Instead, a hungry, out-of-control "bread monster" took over her brain. She discovered that she was motioning him to **"come quickly,"** and asked for **"...more butter and be sure to bring another basket ... please!"** To add insult to injury, Evelyn discovered that she was nearly wolfing the bread down, **"as if it were the only part of the meal that I would have for days."** Embarrassed, she smiled painfully as she recalled it. Predictably, Evelyn ate more than she wanted to eat when both the salad and the entrée arrived.*

Eating slowly might have allowed Evelyn to decide to eat just one slice of bread or a cracker, while enjoying conversation or just appreciating the ambience of the room. It's not about deprivation; it is all about evaluating your choices in connection with your goals and values.

Frequency and Duration of Eating

The frequency with which you eat makes a difference. Are you always putting something to eat in your mouth? Is it a way of filling time?

Many people have reported that not only did frequent eating serve as an unconscious companion to mindless activities, but having a particular taste in the mouth often became habitual and compulsive. Planning ahead for small portions of low fat, healthy snacks such as fresh fruit or raw veggies can chase away hunger sensations, particularly if a meal is delayed. Fresh water or seltzer will satisfy a feeling of emptiness as well.

Remember that you want to slowly and purposefully shrink the size of your stomach, so that you will feel comfortable rather than full when you eat small amounts.

The duration or length of time spent eating is an important factor in winning your weight war. Eating small portions of food is preferable to eating large meals one or two times a day, as your stomach can be stretched when you eat large amounts of food.

Dennis:

Dennis was thirty-eight, but looked as if he were over fifty years old. He weighed well over three hundred pounds. Dennis reported that he could not understand why he didn't "lose" weight when he only ate "one meal a day." What he neglected to say at the time was that the one meal he ate lasted from 5:30 p.m. when he arrived home to 10:30 p.m., just before he went to bed. When I pressed him to record what he ate, he admitted that his daily meal consisted of several helpings of meat, succotash, potatoes, coleslaw, as well as dessert. When I referred him to a nutritionist for some education about starches and fats, he was shocked to discover that his "continuous" meal was adding to his weight. He had to redefine his eating preferences to those of eating small portions of food at specific intervals throughout the day. He had a breakthrough when he discovered that small portions would satisfy him more completely. Moreover, Dennis realized that he was significantly less hungry during the day when he ate breakfast, a nice lunch and a small dinner.

Summary:

For many Americans, sensations of hunger are as much psychological as physical. It's important to become conscious of signals that seem to be responses to stress, emotional turmoil, or an internal conflict. If you can differentiate between those and the specific, physical sensations of hunger, you will have a better idea of the alternatives that might satisfy what is really needed.

One good way of ensuring that you know what normal hunger feels like is to pay attention to your internal sensations after a twelve-hour fast. For example, if you have eaten dinner at 6:00 in the evening, and don't eat again until 6:00 in the morning, then you have fasted for twelve hours. The sensations you feel before you have breakfast is what appropriate hunger feels like.

If you eat only the quantity of food that is represented by your fist, you will ensure that your stomach maintains its natural size. Stop eating at that point to be victorious in your battle of the bulge.

Eating slowly is a wonderful mechanism to evaluate how close to feeling "comfortable" you are. It also increases your satisfaction of what you are eating, so that one forkful of food, eaten mindfully, slowly and consciously, will feel as satisfying as four of them, eaten quickly. The following chapter explores your personal values and unique motivational styles as they impact your eating patterns.

CHAPTER 6

Strategy Five: Goals and Values

Let's be real. No one has any problem being motivated to do something they really want to do! The challenge is to determine how you know that the outcome is worth all the effort that it will take to accomplish it.

Setting goals focuses on how to get what you <u>want</u>. It is not related to pushing yourself hard and feeling unsatisfied; or to saying *unrealistic*, positive things to yourself in the mirror when the mirror is likely to respond, "Who are you kidding?"

It has often been quoted that a "mid-life career crisis is the effect of finding that the ladder of success you have been climbing all these years has been leaning against the wrong wall."

Motivation to achieve a goal relates to being influenced to do what has to be done to accomplish your desired outcome. Problems tend to come up in situations and contexts where people are *told* what to do

A story Abraham Lincoln was fond of telling illustrates this. A frog was mired in a deep, muddy wagon track. His frog friends came by and tried everything they could to encourage him to get out. He hopped on one foot. Then he hopped on the other. He climbed up one side, then the other—continually sliding back down. And try as hard as he might, he just couldn't do it. Finally, at the end of the day, the other frogs gave up hope and left. The next morning they found their frog friend sitting on the lily pad in the pond, looking chipper, joyful, and very pleased with him-

self. His friends asked, "How did you get here? You said you couldn't get out of that rut."

Replied the frog, "I couldn't; but a wagon was coming ... and I had to. I jumped!"

Values:

Values are those principles, convictions, or beliefs that really matter. They work to guide important choices in life, in business and in personal relationships. They give direction and intensity to your motivation when your behavior is in harmony with your values. For example, if you value the advantages of wearing a size 10 dress, this will matter more to you than eating quantities of high calorie foods. You'll change your behavior by eating those proteins, fruits, vegetables which will support your values, and help your body achieve the goals you set. Establishing specific evidence that your values are honored lets you know that you are succeeding.

As you recognize all of the ways your goal weight is important to you, you acknowledge your most important values about how you look, what you weigh, and how you feel inside your body. These values determine your motivation to take action to make it happen. You have personal integrity when your values are in sync with your behavior. For example, if your personal appearance is important to your sense of self-worth, then you will feel depressed when you don't look the way you want to look. Your esteem will increase substantially as you take positive action to achieve what you want. If eating sweet foods has more influence in your life, and temptations are more urgent and important than getting to your weight goals, they will take priority in your food choices.

Lorraine:

Lorraine is a forty-six-year-old mother of three, who has been married for nineteen years to a very slender husband, who she describes as "the most terrific person in the world". According to Lorraine, he doesn't understand why she is overweight because, as he reminds her frequently, they basically eat the same things. It was very discouraging because nothing she had done to reduce her weight seemed to work. Lorraine had given in to negative thoughts, which continually "led her into temptation".

Compromises and Budgets

There are always compromises to make in life. If you choose an expensive dress, you might have to give up purchasing two pairs of slacks. The same is true with a calorie budget. If you are conscientious about reducing excess weight, you will want to limit the number of fat or high carbohydrate calories you consume, as well as the frequency with which you consume them.

It's not about *never*. It is rather about making choices in the interest of winning more important outcomes. Eat high calorie foods cautiously and sparingly, or you will weigh considerably more than you do now. You are probably eating more food now than your body needs in order to stay at your present weight. If you only ate a quantity of food that is consistent with being at your goal weight, you would begin reducing your weight immediately. Translate that to mean small portions so your stomach does not stretch.

Overcoming Challenges

Recall other times in your life when you demonstrated your commitment to overcome challenges to achieve results that were worth your effort. Think about several examples of your success: **How did you do it? What did you say to yourself that helped in your success? How did it feel inside?** It's like inoculating yourself to be more resistant to temptation. You are mentally rehearsing what you will do in the future to be as successful as you were in the past to challenge negative images or thoughts. You can also recognize those positive messages that you need to hear to know you are on the right track. An easy way to do this is to remind yourself of all the benefits that you will have when you are successful. This reinforces your strength and commitment to reduce any temptations and sabotages.

> *Lorraine had faithfully kept a log about what she ate, and recorded how she felt just before she ate it. Lorraine focused on three questions as she kept her log. Making these observations helped her to become aware of self-defeating thoughts or those behavioral triggers that resulted in overeating.*

1. *"Thinking about the situations that are the most difficult for you to control, what are the common points or issues that discourage you from eating responsibly?"*

> *This was another part of the mind game for Lorraine. She discovered that she was least in control later at night when she was tired, lonely, and most vulnerable. She also felt unable to control her eating when she was with family members who could be critical of her attempts to set boundaries on her food choices.*

2. "What happens in connection with food that makes you feel regretful, guilty, or ashamed?"

> Lorraine experienced guilt and shame every night that she snacked after dinner. The irony is that the experience of guilt did not kick in before she engaged in the overeating behavior, and might very well have prevented it.

3. "What behaviors would be signals that you are in control of your weight and your life?"

> Lorraine did not yet understand specifically how she would know she was on target to get to her goal. All of her other "goals" had been met with bitter disappointment and a sense of helplessness; certainly not with any sense of being in control. I validated this as an opportunity to develop a state of curiosity to discover what being in control would be like. That seemed to connect with Lorraine's sense of "fun" to imagine that being in control would be a very different experience from what she anticipated.

Commitment Assessment Questionnaire

Answering the following questionnaire for yourself will bring this dedication into a meaningful framework for you, so you can evaluate your own personal commitment. Appendix II includes these questions as part of the Goal Weight Questionnaire. As an example of how this works, you can trace Lorraine's adventures in exploring her commitment struggles.

1. In your mind, what is something in your life that you wanted to do very much—*and achieved*—even if it took you a long time? If you have had no experience with a long-term commitment, imagine what one would be and how it would feel when it would be accomplished.

> *"I worked very hard to progress in my job since I only had a high school education. I enrolled in community college courses to learn new computer skills; I worked overtime so I would receive good performance reviews, and volunteered to take on some training responsibilities that no one else wanted. I was promoted with good pay raises three times."*

2. How did you decide that was something you wanted to do? Did you discuss it and talk about it? This focuses on the perceived value of the outcome. How did you know it was worth doing?

> *"I wanted to make enough money that would help my family achieve financial security and to have my family be proud of me. I did discuss it all with my husband, and he was fully supportive."*

3. How did it feel inside to want it so much? Notice the sensations and emotions that let you know that the outcome had value for you.

> *"I felt very settled inside with no sense of doubt. It was a warm, comforting feeling that I was doing all that I could."*

4. What was the evidence to you that you were successful? What images did you make in your mind's eye about achieving that goal? What did you say to yourself to get you motivated and excited to do whatever was necessary?

"Every time I received a promotion and a raise, I knew I was being successful. That was exactly what I had imagined and hoped might happen as a result of my hard work."

5. Did you ever become discouraged from reaching that outcome? Was it worth all that work? What kept that determination going?

"The evenings with my family that I gave up to work overtime were very hard on everybody. If I had not had lots of encouragement from my husband that he appreciated my efforts, I would have given up."

6. As you think about all that effort, are you willing to do it all over again from the beginning? Is there anything about going to all that effort as you reach your goal that would make maintaining the weight once you have reached it easier than having to do all that work again? This would protect you against potential relapse.

"Oh my goodness, I don't think I would want to go through that whole thing again. I have worked too hard to start over. It's easier to build on what I already have."

7. What is something that you absolutely would never put inside your body—something that you would be proud to keep out of your body? How do you know, or have a feeling from the bottom of your heart, that you would never do that to yourself? Establish your limits to reinforce your commitment to winning.

"I would never take illegal drugs. That's a choice that I would be ashamed of. I could never set myself up as an example for my kids if I did that."

8. Are there any foods that you absolutely wouldn't eat?

> *"I don't eat, and would never eat coconut, oysters, or eggplant."*

9. Are there any foods that you *want* to put into that category?

> *"I really want to avoid fried foods, donuts, and, I know this sounds silly, but I have a thing for macaroni and cheese."*

10. Ask your future self what kinds of foods *she* would never put in her body.

> *(laughing.) "Gosh, I know she would still never eat coconut, oysters or eggplant. I believe she would not eat fried foods because they are made with fat. She would be very particular, even stingy, about eating sweets, particularly chocolate. I don't think she could ever again be tempted to eat a donut. There might be others, but I can't think of any more right now."*

11. When you go shopping, how do you decide on things you want, that you believe are worth the money it costs?

> *"I know how much I have budgeted to get clothes. I have to work to get the best value I can coordinating colors and styles. They have to be high quality so they can wear well."*

12. Do you feel deprived by limiting yourself to buying things that you can afford? Do you pride yourself on being resourceful about getting the best buy? What will you have to give up in order to have it?—**because you can't always have everything you want at the same moment in time.**

"I really can't afford to feel deprived. I've always had to shop with a restricted budget. It's like a game of making choices. Sometimes, the decisions I make don't always work out the way I thought they would, but I have a good time. I don't take it all so seriously".

Motivational Styles

Everyone has unique experiences in accomplishing goals effectively. It's helpful to think about the different motivational approaches as a range of possibilities rather than an either-or category. That being said, there are several strategies that seem to be more helpful than others to create enthusiasm, commitment and success in reaching your goal weight.

Motivational styles are the personal preferences that filter your perceptions and choices. You habitually use these built-in, intuitive filters to determine **how** you respond to situations in life. These are useful ways of understanding the ideas about how to get motivated effectively. The following five concepts seem to have the greatest impact on the potential for success in winning the weight war. (Note that many people do not fit neatly into the extremes of these categories, but rather include smatterings of everything in between.)

'Carrot or Stick'

'Carrot' people are goal-oriented and reward-driven to look towards positive outcomes and goals they believe are worth having. It is for this motivational type that we create the "future self" to whom you can commit and feel empowered to bring to reality. **'Stick'** folks are motivated to avoid loss, discomfort or distress. They are driven to avoid the negative consequences of remaining overweight or not succeeding in getting what they want. Avoiders are very motivated to distance themselves from being heavy or fat. If they think that eating sweet foods will add to their weight, they avoid these foods at all costs. They are good at noticing difficulties and predicting and solving problems in advance. On the other hand, when they don't create a specific objective for themselves, avoiders can become easily discouraged. Procrastination is a natural consequence when one doesn't do something until it *must* be done or a deadline is looming in order to avert an even more negative consequence. The "carrot" or goal-seeking people often have a hard time doing difficult things that are not as pleasant as looking forward to attaining the objective. "Stick" or avoidant people often have to wait until their situation gets so bad, that staying where they are seems worse than moving forward.

Having a good mix of both of these strategies is probably the most effective motivator of all. It is important to have a specific objective to work towards as well as an avoidance of eating high calorie foods that would add more weight (*which you don't want*). An exercise that will let you encourage the inclusion of both is to make a list of all the benefits of being at your goal weight. Then make an equally long list of all the negatives you associate with maintaining your present weight. Evaluate which of these lists seems to have more energy and influence attached to it. Remember there is nothing inherently good or bad about any of these styles. The more you know and understand them, the more you will be in control.

> *Diane described her goals and objectives very specifically, using positive language regarding all the advantages and benefits that she was looking forward to when she was at her goal weight. It was important for her to generate an avoidance strategy to prevent relapsing into temptation. She would look at a photo*

of herself at her heaviest to remind her of what hap-
pened when she overate, or ate the wrong things.

By comparison, Carol was definitely a person
who motivated herself by focusing almost exclusively
on avoiding what she did not want. Her biggest chal-
lenge was to generate a positive image of her future
self. She spent time imagining the advantages of
buying and wearing clothes which fit her well; show-
ing off her new waist, hearing compliments, and en-
joying the beach.

'Internal' or 'External' Focus of Awareness

Each of us has an awareness of sensations, thoughts, and images, which is generated internally. To the extent that you rely on your **internal** awareness to make decisions, you can effectively evaluate signals of hunger on the one hand, and how you can tell when you have eaten enough to remain healthy and comfortable, on the other. This is consistently the most reliable cue to know when to stop eating. People who rely mainly on **external cues, comments, or the opinions of other people** need an *external* indicator or control factor to help make decisions about how much they have eaten. If you can recognize that the size of a normal stomach is approximately equivalent to one fist, you can use that image or thought as an external cue to think about the volume of food your stomach will hold. External cues such as the numbers on your bathroom scale, seeing how your clothes fit, or even hearing encouraging comments from friends about how well you look are important validations that you are on the right track. Remember that winning this war requires a lifestyle change rather than a simple battle tactic.

Pay attention to how you feel when you are hungry, particularly first thing in the morning after a 12 hour fast. It's not accidental that the term for this meal is "break-fast". Eat slowly, and stay conscious or *mindful* of what you are eating as you focus on recognizing when you feel comfortable sensations inside. Stop eating before you feel full. Use your sense of smell to enhance your taste sensations. Take all the time you need to thoroughly enjoy the aroma of the food you eat. This increases your confidence in trusting your internal awareness of comfort.

Eating slowly will help this **mindfulness**. Take small morsels of food with your fork or spoon. Make sure you can smell the aroma of whatever you have chosen to taste. Imagine what it will taste like. As you put it in your mouth, and slowly draw the spoon or fork from your lips, you can begin to chew, allowing your taste buds to celebrate whatever herbs, spices, or tastes your tongue and saliva can help you differentiate. As you chew slowly, you can swallow easily the morsels of food and the juices that are released. After each bite, close your eyes to focus your attention on how comfortable you are. The slower you go, the more easily you will be able to make these internal judgments.

> *Diane was very external in her approach to eating. She liked being part of a group, so she succeeded beautifully when she found a partner to exercise with, and who also wanted to have company in shopping for food.*
>
> *Carol, on the other hand, enjoyed the challenge of knowing inside when she was full. She celebrated when she could feel how differently her clothes fit her, and she used her future self effectively as her best ally and partner in her battle.*

Options or Procedures

You can make a pretty good guess that those who focus on options are all about having **choices**: what, how much, how often, and where to eat. Then they make decisions based on the specific criteria that define their outcomes. Those who prefer procedures like to have the **structure** that defines the steps necessary to be successful. They are more likely to be motivated by things they "should" do, or believe they "need" to do. Those people who favor the filter of procedures as a way of operating in the world generally want to have an indication of proven results. Then they can commit themselves comfortably to use that structure as the necessary tool to achieve success. They may "audition" or "try out" diet structures until they find one that fits, but they want the step-by-step discipline of a proven structure to guide their eating decisions. People with either of these motivational styles have success in managing their weight as long as they recognize and honor their preferences. To the extent that you can incorporate the elements of the alternative preference, you can have even more opportunity for a wider range of success.

> *Annie was the "poster child" for an options-oriented person. She loved having the privilege of choices and selections of foods. She looked at the idea of controlling the portion size as her "permission" to eat small helpings of anything she wanted, so she never felt deprived.*
>
> *Diane preferred the structured way of thinking about food that Weight Watchers offered. She really connected with the supportive people; and she enjoyed the camaraderie of the weigh-ins. The structure of the food plans made sense to her, and she found it easy to stay committed to it.*

Difference, Progress, or Sameness

This motivational system of filters can influence how encouraged, or discouraged you get as you progress toward your goal. *Each* is helpful at different stages as you fight the battle of your bulge.

A **difference** filter suggests that newness and change are not only acceptable, but are required in order to incorporate a healthy eating strategy, and to maintain interest in achieving the outcome. You need to think about how you need to be eating differently from your present strategy, to make sure you succeed. If you keep the same habits and practice of eating, you will continue to weigh more than you want.

Progress is a mindset that allows you to take on an evaluation of how far you have come, and how far you still have to go. It is a preference for improvement or getting better. As the name suggests, it monitors and evaluates progress toward the goal while maintaining a positive outlook. It defines the "encouragement" element of motivation. This is the structure of your internal cheerleader. You need to reinforce the idea that you are on your way, and can be successful on your journey.

The **sameness** filter operates to ensure that things remain the same. This would mean that people who have this preference do not like to make changes in what, how or how much they eat. This internalized preference for things to remain the same provides the greatest benefit when you have finally reached your goal weight, and are committed to maintaining it.

Past, Present and Future Outlook

The last internal motivation filter that we will focus on is that of an orientation in terms of time frames. For most people, eating is an experience that is *very* focused in the **present:** connecting them with taste, comfort, and satisfaction. Those who overeat tend to forget about the past, often not remembering what they ate several hours before, much less tracking what their eating habits are over a period of several days. The future is ignored or disregarded in favor of present pleasures.

Being successful in winning your personal weight battles requires that you incorporate learning from your past experience and mistakes; recognizing them, and connecting them with the consequences of that behavior. In addition, if you mentally place yourself into your future, you will become conscious of how your food and quantity choices affect your chances of winning. This strategy would eliminate the chronic guilt that often results from overindulging. On the flip side, when you recognize that guilty feelings often occur after you have overeaten or consumed a quantity of higher calorie foods than you intended, you will control those negative emotions by deciding to reject eating those foods. The moment you say "No!" or "No thank you!" to those temptations, you can immediately feel pride and empowerment.

Goals are always future-oriented, even if they are driven by a motivation of avoidance. They are created with regard to honoring your values and motives. The following are guidelines to make goals energized, realistic and ultimately achievable.

Guidelines for Setting Successful Goals

1. **Describe goals in positive language, and reserve negative language for the dangers of maintaining present habits:** "I want to be slender because I will have pride in myself. If I continue to eat chocolate, I won't be able to look good in a bathing suit this summer." Turn any "not's" about your goals into "what do I want instead?" Otherwise you will tie yourself up in "knots". When you assert your commitment

to getting to your objective, you can understand how you will
be enhanced and empowered.

2. **Use specific language:** What do you want to weigh -
specifically? What benefits will you see when you have
reached that weight? By when do you want this goal? At
the very least specify the outcome in terms of a time frame -
weeks, months, or years from now. The more precisely you
can imagine it, the more you will set up the positive self-
talk and internal 'filters' to inspire you. Take into account
there must be a balance of your goals which include personal,
spiritual, and recreational outcomes.

3. **Acknowledge consequences.** Since everything has a price
tag, understand thoroughly what you are getting into. What
is the time commitment? How much effort will be required of
you? What are you likely to give up, **and** is the outcome worth
that effort? Who else will be affected by your decisions, and
how will these important people respond? These questions
evaluate your personal ecology or natural balance in your life.
You want to make sure that all parts of you are in agreement.
If not, you run the risk of self-sabotage.

Donald:

*Donald is a thirty-six-year-old, overweight account
executive whose job required many hours of overtime. He had lapsed into a very inactive lifestyle.
There were many instances where he had to entertain
other business associates both for two- or three-hour
lunches and social occasions with wives, significant
others or just "the guys" from the office. Alcohol was
usually an inherent ingredient of this "social engineering" of his business success. Between writing cor-*

porate reports, frequent traveling, and spending as much time as he could with his family, the ecological issue that Donald faced was to decide which part of his responsibilities would have to be sacrificed so he could be conscientious about a weight-management diet and fitness program. He was unwilling to sacrifice the career he loved and the financial security it offered to him and his family. Donald was looking at it as a polarized issue, like night and day, rather than how to integrate those healthy behaviors into his continuing obligations to further his career.

The solution rested in achieving balance in his life. Donald recalled his college days, when he juggled classes, an outside job, collegiate athletics, and a social life that was adequate enough for him to meet, date, and finally marry the woman of his dreams. What would he have been willing to sacrifice back then, knowing what he knows now? Of course, you could accurately predict that he would give up nothing!

Now was the opportunity to be creative! How many hours a week would he be willing to devote to physical fitness? Donald laughingly recalled how much he loved working out in the college gym. He wanted to work out four times a week. (Not that he actually thought he would be able to pull it off!) We then discussed the various benefits his company offered their executives. Donald admitted that he did not have to punch in with a time clock. He could go to a full gym a couple of miles from his home early in the morning before work, or after work. There was a shower, steam room and sauna there, so he could leave for the office from the gym. He could even take an hour off from time to time to run personal errands or go to children's functions at their school. So Donald could certainly take time off to tend to his own health. After all, since the company had taken out an insurance policy on him as a "key executive", they definitely valued his health and well being.

On social occasions, Donald saw he had an option to choose menu items that were low in calories, or have the sauces, dressings, or gravies put on the side. He could order a bottle of wine and choose to take a small amount for a toast, nurse a glass throughout the evening, or not take any at all. We discussed the potential repercussions of an illness such as diabetes, which would intensely affect his eating and entertaining habits. He agreed that if that were the case, he would have to modify how he lived his life. The conclusion he reached was that if he could make it work because he had to, he could also be successful because he wanted to accomplish this goal.

4. **Criteria of success.** This marks out the evidence that you use to confirm that you have accomplished your goal. The number of pounds that are measured by your scale gives you objective data. More important are what sensations will you be experiencing when celebrating our victories. Exactly what will you hear, see or feel when you know you have reached your goal? What would an observer see, hear and feel at that moment?

5. **Identify your personal internal resources.** List and appreciate your qualities, skills and energies that will aid you in achieving your goals. For instance, being *determined, persistent, and enthused* will help in reminding you that anything worth doing is worth the effort that it takes to make it work. Being rebellious will help you chart your own independent course. Stubbornness will get you over the hump of the certain challenges you will encounter. Who are the people who could assist you or mentor you to achieve your goals? Are there any people who can serve as your role models?

6. **Take personal responsibility:** Get proactive. Being in control of your weight is **your** responsibility to fulfill. *You* will have to make it happen. You can dream, wish, or hope that you will win the lottery, and will never have to work again, *but that's a fairy tale.* The reality is that the world rarely lets anything fall in your lap. Make an action plan, breaking a big goal into realistic, smaller steps which you can easily recognize as you accomplish each one. For example, you may have to restrict intake of calories by **only** 500 a day, and increase exercise to an hour a day so that you are burning off another 500 calories. At the end of a week, you will have reduced your weight by two pounds. In only five weeks, you will have taken off ten pounds. This may not be a great deal in the large scheme of things, but it proves that you are capable of accomplishing this feat. Mentally rehearse having that goal in your future as thoroughly as possible.

7. **Be flexible in formulating plans to reflect reality appropriately.** One of the main reasons people don't succeed in gaining their outcomes is that they get discouraged when

things don't work out as planned. If what you are doing is not working, do something else.

Ineffective strategies to create outcomes that will actually work are similar to the stereotype of an "ugly" American traveling in France. **"Where is the train station?"** he asks.

The native replies, *"Je ne comprend pas."* ("I don't understand.") Then, **very slowly**, in his best French accent, the American asks again, **"Where ees ze t-r-a-i-n st-a-sh-onn?"** (It didn't work any better the second time either.)

8. **Remember to appreciate yourself when you have made even small advances and goals.** We all spend entirely too much time being self-critical and not nearly enough time expressing self-appreciation that directs needed positive energy inside. It provides appropriate courage to continue in the desired direction. This is what *encouragement* is all about.

There are several effective strategies for achieving success that re-program our mindset, determination, expectations, and choices about the best way to realize those expectations. The concept of the **"Mental Rehearsal for Success"** is an effective mechanism to tap into your history of successes, and explores how you actually formulated that structure in your mind. In order to understand how to do this for yourself, you need some information about "submodality distinctions" which reduce your internal experience down to the basic sub-qualities of **seeing, hearing and feeling:** the components of your experience. (This is included in Appendix III)

Summary:

Self-motivation is the significant factor in winning your struggle to control your weight. Motivation is based on honoring your highest values and aligning your behavior to match them. Identifying those values is the first step. Discovering the actions and behaviors that honor those values is the next one. Having limits, boundaries, budgets, and choices in life are necessary components of a balanced existence. We all live inside of these limits, and make the best of the "hand we are dealt."

Sometimes we forget our past successes in overcoming blocks, sabotages, as well as temptations. We need to recall our history of being determined, positive, and empowered to be in control.

The self-assessment questionnaire gives you insight into your resources and personal commitment.

Motivational styles are the personal preferences that filter your decisions. They tend to be unconscious; therefore all the more powerful. The highlighted preferences seem to be the most influential in determining how successful you are in reducing excess weight. Perhaps you will notice that each end of the spectrum is useful at specific times in the weight control process.

The motivational preference filters are: Carrot / Stick, Internal / External, Options / Procedures, Differences / Progress / Sameness, or even Past / Present / Future

It is important to:

1. Describe goals in positive language, and reserve negative language for the dangers of maintaining present habits.

2. Use specific language.

3. Acknowledge consequences, and establish appropriate criteria of success.

4. Identify your personal internal resources.

5. Take personal responsibility.

6. Be flexible in formulating plans to reflect reality appropriately.

7. Remember to appreciate yourself when you have made even small advances and goals

Mindful consciousness is a key concept in controlling your awareness of what you eat, how much you eat and how satisfying that food is. Chapter Seven explores how to use your highest values to protect your commitment from habitual temptations and sabotages created by emotional eating responses. You will discover how clinical hypnosis can train your higher consciousness and automatic response system to make progress in weighing what you want.

CHAPTER 7

Strategy Six: Defeating Sabotages and Temptations

Why do I eat when I know I am not even hungry? This question is the most relevant and important question that plagues everyone who struggles with her weight. Those who are in control of their weight value the idea of **"Eating to Live"**. As a group, they pay more attention to how food nourishes their body. **"Living to Eat"** seems to be a main focus of attention for those who are overweight. It is driven by "emotional eating" and occurs when food becomes the main channel of emotional nourishment and well-being.

To take a page out of David Letterman's comedic banter, the following are the "Top Ten" emotional needs that drive overeating:

10. **Social temptation:** wanting to be part of a group. This goes as far back as Adam and Eve – and a certain apple!

9. **Eat until you're full:** – a member of the "clean plate club." After all, the poor children in India or Africa would love a care package made up of the food on your plate you don't want. I never did figure out how they would know if I cleaned my plate or not! No care packages were ever sent from my house.

8. **Mindless activity** – keeping your hands busy. Eating really takes very little business. It's not like typing, painting, crosswords, cross-stitch, knitting, (or even playing Wii),

7. **Regret and disappointment** over past actions - wishing things would be different. Of all the people

who have told me that this is a trigger for eating when they aren't even hungry, none have said that it helps. The regret is still there – even after they eat!

6. **Happy celebrations** when depriving yourself of sweet food is unthinkable. Just think of how you can make up for all that happiness when you are full of regret for eating fattening foods!

5. **Anger** with other people or situations. Ditto the last two observations – only **you** can get angry at yourself instead of others.

4. **Frustration over lack of control** or to change the circumstances or results. Lack of control is what happens to you when you decide to overeat.

3. **Guilt** or perceived responsibility for behavior. Get the guilt over eating fattening foods before you eat them – then you can avoid it.

2. **Response to stress** and trauma. You will provide additional stress for yourself when you can't fit into your clothes.

1. **And the number one emotional problem that drives overeating is: ... anxiety.** It's just misplaced. Be afraid – be very afraid of putting more weight on than your metabolism can handle.

I am sure there are others, but these are the most common reasons that I have heard over the years. What is interesting to observe is that the higher the intensity or emotional content of the need, the more that one eats high calorie, sweet, "comfort" foods. Let's examine each in turn, and then look at some alternatives:

Social Temptation: wanting to be part of a group.

You can be a part of a group in many ways even if eating is involved. First, you are the only one in actual control of what gets put in your mouth. When the crowd suggests going out for pizza, you always have the choice to order a salad, and then share in only one piece of pizza. You could order a beverage, and keep the rest of the group company while they eat more fattening choices. They are not mutually exclusive. You can put social connection and participation in the context of maintaining important ties, while still being true to your commitment to getting your weight goals.

Eating Until Full

Many people believe that they have to be "full" to justify when to stop eating. When you were a little baby and went to sleep with a full tummy, your body used that nutrition efficiently and effectively as you grew physically and mentally at a rapid rate. As you reached your adult height, your metabolism began to slow down. The only growth then moved from an increase in height to an increase in girth. Not a good idea! 'Clean Plate Clubs' were demanded or encouraged by worried parents who wanted to make sure their children were well-nourished. You can't eat in the same way you used to eat as a young person – nor can you use those familiar strategies to determine when to stop eating.

Many people believe that if they don't eat until they are "full to bursting" they are not getting enough to eat. The main challenge is to remind yourself that unless you control food portions to total a "fist-full" of food, you will continue to eat more calories than your body can efficiently process. It takes time for this new way of thinking to become a habit. If you fall "off the wagon", so to speak, get right back on with a renewed determination.

Mindless Activity (keeping your hands busy)

The television is on, and the kids want microwave-popped popcorn. Suddenly you discover that the movie is only half over, and you have already started on the second bowl. Your co-worker brought in a large bag of M&Ms or pretzels which are served in an elegant glass dish, and put it out for all to share. It starts out with just a small handful, but you find yourself going back for more – and more. You probably can't recall eating or even getting any pleasure from eating..

The solution is somewhat simplistic, but is very effective to help stop mindless eating. Plan what you want to eat every day, and bring your own food in with you to work. This is the principle behind the "lunch-box" psychology discussed in the eleventh chapter. Be purposeful, and decide when and where you want to have a snack and measure out a small portion. You might even interrupt the habitual behavior by standing up rather than stay seated when you eat. Stop engaging in any other activity whether it is watching TV, reading or even talking on the phone, etc. Eat the snacks *very* slowly and be mindful of the chewing, the taste and enjoying your treat, so that you are consciously aware of consuming it. When your planned snack is consumed, sit back down to enjoy the rest of the movie, the television show, or get back to work.

Regret and Disappointment (or wishing things would be different)

Everyone has moments they want to have back, especially with hindsight being twenty-twenty. Sorry – it isn't going to happen, regardless of how much food you eat. Face whatever issue is going on in the present. Determine how is your present, (or possible future) being impacted by those regretted events. Look for the lessons you learned, as well as ways to repair any damage done; then move on. If you continue to look over your shoulders at the past, you won't be able to look out for opportunities in the future. When you accept yourselves in spite of all your mistakes (or maybe because of them) you let go of the regret, and give yourself peace of mind. Recognize all the changes in your life you have already made, and all the ways you have personally benefited from those changes. You can empower yourself to make lifestyle changes in the future, regardless of those negative experiences in the past.

Happy Celebrations (depriving yourself of sweet food is unthinkable)

Life goes on. You can't, and won't stop living just because you are battling the bulge. Celebrations, happy events, or special times with people you love and appreciate are to be enjoyed. You can plan for these events, so you can enjoy yourself without feeling deprived. I truly believe in the concept of **"Five steps forward toward your goal – one step back to enjoy the side trips."** If you know you will be attending a big event, be *very* disciplined for two weeks before, and a week afterwards. While you are there, continue to be mindful of taking small portions, while sampling everything you want. (Be a gourmet!) Remember to thoroughly enjoy yourself. You can use this concept to maintain motivation and commitment because "all the weight of the

fear of deprivation" is lifted. You can be more in control of your life –
and enjoy it thoroughly.

Anger (with other people or situations)

Anger and resentment takes away more of your own internal energy
than they do from those who are the object of your resentment. When
you eat while you are angry, you can't digest the food well. Eating does
not fix any problem. It only adds regret and guilt about overeating, not
to mention adding those additional calories. The recipient of these
more complex emotions is you! Decide how long you will allow the
anger to dominate your thoughts; then get busy evaluating plans to
remedy the problem. Are these plans realistic? Will they effectively
solve the problem? Are they in your power to accomplish? Who else
can you recruit to help you solve any problem you face?

> *Carol had expressed a great deal of anger at her par-*
> *ents and grandmother for being demanding and*
> *critical. She felt helpless to change the environment*
> *in which she was raised. Anger was now being di-*
> *rected at her own body by eating "comfort foods" with*
> *large amounts of fat and calories, even though she*
> *knew the overeating was causing her to weigh more*
> *than she wanted. Carol focused her efforts on iden-*
> *tifying healthy alternatives to express this anger, such*
> *as writing letters to each of her parents, listing all of*
> *her resentments. The important thing to remember is*
> *that these letters were **never** mailed. The important*
> *healing came from having written them. Carol could*
> *then begin to move forward to gain control of her*
> *weight, independently of any anger.*

Frustration over Lack of Control

Feeling frustrated when things don't seem to go the way you want is the ultimate definition of stress. It is difficult to stay calm when your expectations and plans are shattered. Control seems out of reach. It seems like the only thing you have control over is what you eat. The good news is that you are the only one who has absolute control over what you eat. So you can still honor your commitments to yourself about what you put into your mouth.

Many people work in stressful environments. There is always pressure to perform at ongoing higher levels of excellence and efficiency. Being calm is a state of mind. It is important to focus on your breathing, taking slow breaths all the way in, and releasing the breath twice as slowly. More oxygen can get to your brain, and you can more clearly think through your options. Embrace the concept of taking a "mental vacation" for two or three minutes to interrupt your stress spiral.

Guilt (perceived responsibility for behavior)

Guilt is a necessary emotion, in that it lets you know that you did something that violated your own value system in some way. It is a signal that you need to bring your behavior back in line with your values. (It's also a good indication that you are not a sociopath, who experiences no guilt over bad behavior.) Acknowledging responsibility, making amends for actions, and asking forgiveness are three effective steps to relieve legitimate guilt.

Most of the time, guilt is misplaced and unnecessary. Guilt tends to be imposed by others to cover up insecurities, judgments, or criticisms. Even if the guilt is deserved because you have made a mistake, eating certainly does not make it better. It only complicates the problem by adding overweight to it.

Responses to Stress

The reason that certain events are stressful and traumatic is that they are unexpected. Their impact is always negative, and the degree of control over them is minimal. In addition to the previous suggestion to generate a state of comfort and relaxation, you can recall a time when you felt competent, confident, and handled unexpected or complicated events with ease and self-assurance. If you did it once, you will be able to do it now. It reinforces your competency to handle life's challenges. In order for you to be motivated to read this book, and to make changes in your life, you have indeed had many experiences of competence and confidence. For many, these experiences are discounted or disregarded. Overeating only overwhelms you with **more** of what you want to get rid of – and gives you additional problems.

Anxiety (the number one problem that drives people to overeat or eat sweet "comfort" foods)

Anxiety is caused by "what if" worries that are focused on a future that is, by definition, unknown to us. The fact that this future is unknown is what makes life such an adventure. You never experience anxieties about things which have passed. You already know what happened. It's like hearing a bad joke for the *second* time. Food becomes an attempt to replace and diminish anxiety with something akin to comfort. After all, we are hard-wired from our birth to find food and a "full tummy" satisfying and comforting. Even harsh or emotionally neglectful parents had to feed their children. (Otherwise they would not have survived.) For many, that food became the only expression of love that they had experienced. It is an understandable knee-jerk response to search out food when stressed, hurt or anxious. There are other strategies to manage anxiety. Following are some suggestions.

Transform anxiety into curiosity

Another concept of not knowing the future, but which is considered more pleasant is curiosity. You can remember seeing a wrapped present with your name on it, and will find yourself intensely curious about what is in it. If you think about it, it's almost more fun to wonder about the contents than to tear the wrapping open and discover what it is. Both anxiety and curiosity are states of **not knowing,** but curiosity is a much more pleasant state of mind.

Anxiety serves as a signal that you need emotional comfort and reassurance. Most people can relate to the experience of comforting a young child who has skinned her knee, sees blood, and becomes anxious that blood means that she will die. You can give her comfort and reassurance to that child, because you have the wisdom and experience to know that she will survive. Washing it gently, putting a bandage on it, and giving that knee a little kiss is **all** she needs to get back out and play. The same is true for the very scared part of you. Eating to relieve anxiety will give you a **certainty**: that **you will** put additional weight on.

New ways of relieving stress

Realizing and honoring the specific cause of your hurt, angry, sad, or scared feelings will determine the most effective relief for them. For example, if you're lonely, find new ways of connecting with interesting people. You could volunteer to help an organization, take a course which would interest you, or go to social events. Just don't eat to relieve loneliness or stress. Eating is a poor substitute for human companion-ship. If you are being treated unfairly or disrespected by others, it is sometimes necessary to find the courage, strength and resolve to con-front mistreatment. It is important to learn about assertiveness skills which will teach you to maintain your own self-respect while you are standing up for your rights.

Honor the positive needs (while shifting the negative behaviors)

It is important to create more effective and efficient ways of satisfying the positive intentions of those internal needs that produce symptoms simulating hunger. There are many ways of thinking about the force or emotional needs that seem to drive your practice of eating even when you are not hungry, eating too much at one time, or eating fat-tening foods. The way I like to think of it is to formulate a metric or percentage. ***"Out of 100 percent, identify the percentage of you that wants to get to your goal weight and to maintain it there."*** If 100 percent is the answer, there should be nothing stopping you from win-ning this war on your weight. More often than not, you will recognize that while the major percentage of you values all the benefits you have acknowledged of reaching your goal weight, there is a smaller **'part'** of you which has important concerns. These psychological concerns or intentions are always positive in the context of getting important out-comes on your behalf. If they are not honored and effectively satisfied in other ways, these intentions will be powerful enough to sabotage even the strongest good intentions. Consequently you will continue to use the only habitual response that you know: over-eating. Once you can identify the psychological and emotional needs that over-eating attempts to serve, you can focus on all the potential alternatives which will satisfy all these important needs.

Viable Options

This is where reality and possibility merge. Because you are a creative, resourceful person, you are able to imagine creating a "laundry list" of viable options which would satisfy those needs at least as effectively as eating. These options will go from the most trivial and imaginative to the most useful and practical. You can imagine that this internal "part" of you which had been producing that overeating behavior could select which of those options would be the most appropriate in the circumstances that you face every day. This is an adaptation of the NLP intervention, "Six Step Reframe", created by Richard Bandler and John Grinder, which establishes appropriate alternative behaviors to satisfy those internal needs. For example:

> **Grace:**
>
> *Grace is thirty-seven years old, the newly-divorced mother of two sons in middle school, who was getting back into the swing of her career. She had to balance her work responsibilities with her role as "supermom" since Dad was no longer in the picture. As she was committed to being competent, efficient, and successful, she felt bombarded and overwhelmed by the amount of responsibility at work and her anxiety in response to it. With all this added stress, she put on nearly 40 pounds.*
>
> *While the work environment itself was stressful, Grace and her coworkers shared many personal concerns, worries, aggravations, and victories be-*

tween and amongst themselves all in an "eating" en-
vironment at lunch and breaks. Everyone brought in
homemade sweets and baked goods to share "to sweet-
en up the sour notes." Lunch was available at work,
but generally consisted of high fat or carbohydrates
like macaroni and cheese, pizza, or fried chicken. It
was important to help Grace develop relevant alter-
natives to overeating.

The old habitual behavior which seems to have control over eating has
outlived its usefulness and has negative consequences. It's very important to recognize, honor, and satisfy those needs and intentions which
generate those eating habits in even more effective ways. Even the
most ill-advised patterns of behaviors can be changed without losing
any of the benefits that they attempt to serve. It becomes a "win-win"
scenario as the negative behaviors are replaced with equally satisfying
positive ones. The following is a transcript of a counseling session
which focuses on finding better ways of honoring those positive needs
and intentions.

"Grace, you may believe that there is nothing positive
in the intentions of this part, because you are so upset
at the effects of that overeating. Everyone moves to-
wards pleasure and away from pain. It's as if a part
of you had generated that eating behavior because it
was attempting to meet some important needs. If you
can identify what those needs are and honor them,
you could find better, more efficient ways of satisfying
those internal needs and serving those positive inten-
tions. Imagine you can step into a state of personal
curiosity and in the most accepting and welcoming
way possible for you, get in touch with the 'part' of

you that generates the inappropriate eating behavior. You want to ask permission of that part to share with you whatever needs or intentions are being served by eating even when you are not hungry. That part has valuable information to share about the positive outcomes it is attempting to get for you. Ignoring this bit of information will result in an active sabotage of even the best laid-out plans.

Yes/no signals

First, you need establish distinct communication signals that differentiate between a "yes" or "true" response to an idea, and another one that indicates a response that means "no" or "wrong" or "false". You want to make sure that all the parts of you will be in agreement with the options and alternatives that will satisfy those needs. You will be checking back from time to time with that part of you that you think is responsible for those overeating behaviors.

Think of a specific time when you felt confident inside that something was true for you; or about which you had no doubt. Notice the internal sensations that let you know that this is true, and pay attention to what you say to yourself.

Pay close attention to the very different physical sensations that you experience inside, and what words come to mind when you know something to be "wrong" or "untrue" for you. Observe the distinctions between these two experiences."

Grace: "True" feels like a comfortable, settled heaviness at the pit of my stomach and I say 'Yes' to myself emphatically. When I believe something to be untrue, there is a tight feeling up in my chest, and I can feel my heart pounding. I can almost feel my head shaking 'No'. The difference is unmistakable."

"Now you can invite the part responsible for the overeating to use these familiar signals to communicate with your conscious awareness. Ask that part if it would be willing to share the positive intentions that are manifested by the overeating behavior. After all, it doesn't occur in a vacuum. Reassure that part that you will honor those needs and positive intentions, and that you will find better ways to satisfy them."

Grace: (After closing her eyes and focusing her awareness internally) "That part of me wants to feel comforted and secure. I have been very lonely, so that when I eat with the group I am close to, I feel like I am accepted as an equal. I get social energy and warm vibrations from my coworkers in the lunch room that I haven't been able to find anywhere else. They have been my only support system when 'the chips are down' I feel if I stopped baking goodies to contribute along with everyone else; or if I didn't eat the treats that my friends brought, it's like a slap in the face to them."

"Wow! That's important. Take some time to appreciate that you have a part of you that really cares *that you feel accepted and have that sense of your own 'social security'. Remind that part that you will do nothing to diminish this part or the important purpose it serves. You want to allow this part to become even more empowered by choosing alternative behaviors other than eating sweets that would satisfy those needs in even more effective ways."*

Grace: "That feels very good inside. That part of me seems at peace with the idea of finding other ways."

"Now, what I want you to do, is to make a connection with that creative unconscious, higher consciousness, or master-mind from which you find your most innovative ideas. Create an extensive 'laundry list' of your best accomplishments, as well as any behaviors that you connect with being confident, and another list which would maintain the social and support connections. These can be used as resources to satisfy those important needs instead of eating."

"Now, ask that 'responsible' part to choose at least three different behaviors from that long list, any one of which would satisfy the needs. Once other behaviors are found which fulfill and gratify those needs and positive intentions, you can resolve all the internal conflict, which could interfere with your commitment to take the weight off, and keep it off."

Grace enjoyed this process thoroughly. To meet the needs of being confident and to relieve stress, she chose to do crossword puzzles, get exercise by going up and down the stairs or walking around the block.

The third option was to take care of her house plants and her garden. She acknowledged that her calm and confident feelings and alternative behaviors were certainly different from being anxious and insecure. The really important need to maintain the social connection at work took the most time to satisfy.

Grace: *"I think my friends might be willing to help me in my efforts as long as I continued to eat with them. It really shouldn't matter to them what I choose to eat. I can even make enough of the low-fat, healthy foods that I prepare for myself to share with them. Maybe it will inspire a couple of the others to join me. We might take breaks together, walking around the building if it's nice out to get a little more exercise. From time to time, I can even take a little taste of their treats. When they know that my intentions are just to reduce my weight rather than to upset them, they should be okay with that. Those options sound good."*

"Now, Grace, invite that responsible part to agree to use those alternative behaviors instead of eating fattening foods exclusively for at least two weeks, to discover how satisfying it is. If ever these are not sufficient for any reason, invite that part to contact the creative energy inside of you to generate even more possibilities that you could decide would be worth doing. As a last check, ask inside if any part of you has any concerns about the changes you made for yourself today."

*Grace focused her attention inside to determine
if there was any part of her that would have any concern or objection to those changes. She took a deep
breath, smiled, and said **"No!"** emphatically.*

Most slender people "eat to live". This means they focus on nourishing their bodies with healthy foods, and they *stop* eating when they feel comfortable rather than stuffing themselves. Food is not the most important focus of their days (or nights). Sometimes, eating itself seems to be nothing more than a necessary distraction from other important activities.

Winning the 'Deprivation' Battle

One of the major detractors to winning your personal weight war is the resistance against possible deprivation of foods you love to eat, and have become used to eating. Nobody likes to be told that they **can't** have things—even if it is for all the right reasons. A part of us rebels. You dig in your heels, eat what you want, then get to "enjoy" all the regret and guilt which follow this rebellion. I happen to like and admire the "little rebel" who inhabits a part of your emotional home. After all, it is this wonderful little rebel who gets upset about your being overweight in the first place. You derive all your unique personality characteristics and preferences from your intense desire to be independent, strong, and in control.

You want to make this little rebel part a strong ally rather than a combatant. "It's not about *never* – it's about using discretion and control in the service of what you desire to achieve."

Satisfying the Inner Rebel

If you ignore the importance of recognizing, honoring and satisfying that part of you that rebels when it develops a yearning for a favorite food, your taste buds simply will not be satisfied with an alternative. As I mentioned earlier, the mindset that would be most helpful is that of becoming a gourmet who is very picky and discriminating about what you eat as well as how much you eat. In the same way that you get into financial trouble if you spend more than you can afford, if you eat more than your body can metabolize or efficiently use as fuel, this excess will be stored as fat. When you restrict the *quantity* of high calorie or high fat foods, you can enjoy the **quality** of the taste sensations you crave without paying the high penalty of excess weight. The little rebel can indeed "have the cake and eat it too." When there is an adequate opportunity to satisfy a taste sensation, the rebel part of you can *appropriately* rebel against being deprived of the benefits of your important long-term outcomes.

Make plans for, and then implement regular relapses. This puts you in control of how often, and how much you "cheat". I truly believe these planned relapses give your life meaning. It makes it much easier to be committed to eating healthy for the remainder of the time. It means that if there is a party, special dinner or celebration, you can reduce the quantity of food the week before the event and for the week following, so you can enjoy the tastes and treats at the party. You will not put on weight, if you remember to limit the quantity of food you eat to that of a fistful, even if that contains a higher number of calories.

Of course there are instances where there is simply no other alternative to developing a "never again" mindset. In the same way that an alcoholic physiologically processes alcohol differently than a social drinker, some people have an intense physiological response to a food. Refusing to eat certain foods is a lifestyle that can become a habit. Vegetarians, or those who must restrict their intake of wheat or milk products, certainly can relate to the wisdom of this decision. Adding excess fat is like an allergic reaction, and must be treated as such, because your body cannot metabolize the food efficiently.

> *Carol was very concerned that once she tasted a little sweet, she would begin to crave more and more of it. It seemed to feed on itself, so to speak. She said emphatically that it was easier to say no the first time rather than taste it and have to battle the craving in addition to the food. That was the only way she could stay in control.*

Uses of Self-Hypnosis to Help Overcome Temptations

There are times when you feel helpless to either recognize or change those ingrained behaviors that expose us to the habitual, eating temptations that result in weight problems. Focusing your awareness on your internal experience will give you an insight into what created those negative habits, as well as an awareness of the options, strategies, and resources that are needed to change those habits. By using clinical hypnosis, it is possible to "reprogram" your internal mental and emotional "software" to influence and determine your eating choices. In addition to working with a mental health professional skilled in hypnosis to guide you in this process, you can learn self-hypnosis to help create or recognize your existing, empowering resources which have the potential to resolve internal conflicts or issues which influence your eating decisions.

To explain further, hypnosis is an internally-focused awareness of your internal experience. It is subjective in that no two experiences are exactly alike, though most people describe it as being calm, comfortable, and relaxed. When you generate this voluntary, relaxed state you are more open to positive suggestions that enhance or reinforce your values or principles. Hypnosis is similar to meditation, guided imagery, day-dreaming; or those in-between moments just before you drop off to sleep or just before you wake up in the morning. You experience a natural, altered state of consciousness when you are immersed in a good book. A good author will weave such a riveting tale, that you are drawn into the background, emotions, dialogue, inner thoughts, and the events that transpire in the story. Although you are certainly aware that you are physically in the here-and-now, as you read the words printed on the page, your imagination can figuratively transport you to another land, seeing inside another character's internal processes or experience as he or she relates to and interprets reality.

For those clients who maintain that they have never been able to relax, you can imagine what it would be like to be on your own private desert island populated only with people who can make you feel safe and secure.

"Close your eyes. Be there, seeing what you see: the shapes, the colors, the scenery, the people who are important to you. Hear the sounds that you hear in that space, as well as noticing what you are saying to yourself as you inhabit this scene. Smell any fragrances or aromas around. Feel the comfortable air around you.... and feel the feelings of comfort and relaxation, safety and security. Focus on the sensations of comfort, relaxation, and security that accompany your imagined experience."

Imagined experiences can thus become as realistic and powerful as memories of actual experiences.

Once you have this personal imagery clearly represented in your mind's eye, think of this as your personal 'Garden of Eden' or paradise.

It can become your Genesis to create an atmosphere of suggestibility from which you can accept positive thoughts and ideas. Self-hypnosis suggestions could be framed in the first person, "I", or in the second person "you," as if you were being encouraged by a loving "cheerleader". A self-hypnosis script that you would personalize to reflect the behavior you want to integrate inside could resemble the following:

A complete script, and guides to using self-hypnosis are included in Appendices VII, VIII and IX. If you prefer a prerecorded CD with this script, you can order one. (Details are in the last section of the book.) Another option is to tape or digitally record the script yourself.

One of the most significant conflicts that many people experience is the fear that by committing to reducing excess weight, they will have to give up things they love. Questions that address these concerns generally take the form of the following:

Can you identify anything positive about being at your present weight that you would want to preserve?

Is there anything that you would miss by being at your goal weight?

Focus on what is important in your life, and remind yourself how achieving your goal weight will help you. What do you need as skills, qualities, interests or abilities you do not yet possess? What would you like to do in your life that you find rewarding and stimulating, if you are not doing it now? How will you know when you get there?

Ammunition for Your War Chest

To win your war, you need all the ammunition available to you in your 'war chest':

➥ Your personal values associated with achieving your desired weight

➥ Believing that you are worth the effort it will take to insure your success

➥ The objective facts such as monitoring what you put in your mouth and relating it to measuring how much you weigh on a regular basis

➥ The advantage of learning from the experiences of others who have been successful

➥ Setting a specific goal, and recognizing how it is important to you

➥ Honoring your own opinions, values, and evidence of success

➥ Engaging in helpful and encouraging comments and self-talk

➥ Focus on shifting negative behaviors, attitudes, or circumstances that prevent you from success to those which would be effective and advantageous to you.

"Overcoming the Temptation Battle", included in its entirety in Appendix VI, is an effective and powerful exercise to remove temptation by interrupting the negative pattern of discouraging thoughts and overcome those automatic habitual behaviors preventing you from avoiding temptations which accompany reaching a plateau when you staying with a program for a long period of time. Once you stop the negative energies and discouraging self-talk, you can remind yourself of all the positive aspects included in your internal "war chest" mentioned above. The advantage of this is that you can engage in this exercise as often as you would like.

When you identify and honor the emotional needs which pull you away from your goals; and find different strategies to satisfy those needs, you are resolving those internal conflicts which stand in the way of winning the war on your weight.

Summary

Emotions are the key internal forces which drive overeating, even when intellectually you know you have eaten enough. While it is important to recognize the major influence of emotions in your personal struggle, it is vital to understand that you can ultimately be in control of how you respond to them.

The top ten emotional triggers seem to be:

1. Social connections,

2. A perceived sensation of fullness as a signal to stop eating,

3. Habitual eating without thought or purpose,

4. Regret over the past

5. Happy celebrations

6. Anger over other people or situations

7. Frustration or lack of control

8. Guilt

9. Responding to stressful events

10. Anxiety

Shifting or changing your attitude, responses, internal dialogue, and behavior will provide the antidotes to negative emotional states. Several of the alternatives are relaxation and slow breathing, staying alert and mindful while you are eating, as well as interrupting the negative images and thoughts so you can refocus on your positive commitments, energies, and objectives. Releasing anger, resentments and regrets from the past allows you to let go of what you can no longer control, and focus on what you will do from this point forward into the rest of your life. A hypnosis script is included to reprogram your internal automatic processes.

Changing limiting beliefs which stop you from reaching your goals is the subject of the next chapter.

CHAPTER 8

Strategy Seven: Win the Battle of Emotional Hunger

It's really important to recognize and identify the kinds of situations which are upsetting to you. Once you can do that, you can begin to create antidotes to the stress or those internal needs that generate the food cravings. This puts you in control of your life and decisions. You can create powerful, positive, internal resources and beliefs that are intense enough to counter the lure of sweet, fattening foods.

Childhood roots

The frustrations that disrupt the commitment to get to your goal weight often have their roots in childhood – a time when you were vulnerable and insecure. This was the onset of negative beliefs about your capacities to be in control of your life, or even deserve to have this control. As we explored in the last chapter, the one symbol of an intimate or emotional connection is food. When a baby cries, even a "bad" mother sticks a bottle of milk in the baby's mouth, regardless of whether that baby is held or even comforted. An early negative self-definition that you believe, replays itself many times throughout your life. This response has become automatic. The food response to mood disruptions has been imprinted or programmed into your "unconscious" software that determines behavior. When negative things continue to happen as part of life, food continues to be reinforced as an object of comfort.

Sabotages and temptations often result from negative beliefs and will derail your mission. Some of these are even created by well-meaning persons who want company while they eat. They say such things as, "Why do you want to be on a diet? You look fine to me. Let's order the fried onion rings and split it."

High Calorie Tastes

Desserts go down so easily, and taste so good, it's hard to believe how many calories and carbohydrates are attached to each of them. But when you exercise hard for twenty minutes and discover that you have only burned off two hundred calories, you might want to think twice or even three times before you eat those high calorie items as you realize how easy it is to add two hundred calories, compared with how difficult it is to burn them off.

Chains of behavior

There are personal "chains" of behavior that seem to automatically link one action to another. These links in the chain take purposeful decisions out of the eating equations.

Abigail goes shopping late in the afternoon on Thursday. Feeling low on energy, she buys a large bag of cookies. As she unloads the groceries, the cookies are the last items to be unloaded, and are put in the front of the pantry cupboard. On Friday, when Abigail gets home from work, she is both tired and hungry. When she goes to the pantry to choose something to eat, the first thing she sees is the bag of cookies in front of any other food. She snacks on the cookies as she starts dinner. By the time dinner is ready, Abigail has already consumed more calories than are in the well-balanced dinner she has planned. No longer hungry, she still wants to eat with her family, and ends up feeling very full. Since she has already sabotaged her intentions, Abigail figures all is lost for the night, scraps her commitment, finishes up the bag of cookies, and goes to bed. In the morning she becomes depressed and guilty because she had 'blown' her pledge by eating those fattening things the night before. As a result, she eats all morning to help herself feel better – and so the vicious cycle continues.

Everyone engages in similar kinds of automatic chains of actions. One strategy which will effectively unravel these chains is to recall the last time that your eating was out of control.

- ➼ Think about the specific triggers that just preceded that eating behavior.

- ➼ What were you thinking, imaging in your mind's eye, and feeling inside your body? (You might want to write these down as you remember them.)

- ➼ Continue tracking these back until you determine the first link in your chain.

- ➼ Create alternative behaviors at each part of the 'chain' which serve the positive purposes and intentions, but which don't involve eating.

- ➼ You can use the internalized future image of how you want to look and feel.

If you want to change your habitual relationship to food, you need to interrupt the sabotage at the times in your life when you feel most vulnerable. You can then create specific suggestions that would be helpful for you to feel more safe, secure, and confident. Think about a time and place in your life when you felt safe, secure, calm, relaxed, and peaceful or any other similar word which represents those kinds of positive, constructive feelings.

Abigail admitted that her fears, frustrations, and disappointments often become so overwhelming that her best intentions are derailed. The example she offered was when her supervisor called her into his office to criticize the month-end report that her team was responsible for writing. Abigail felt insecure and nervous about her ability to succeed on the job. She complained that she was stuffing herself with sweets and breads as the end of each month loomed. To help Abigail recognize and use her internal positive resources to manage her fears, it was important for her to experience times in her life which represented calmness, safety, and confidence.

"As you recall at least three times in your life when you felt safe and secure, pick the best one. Then focus on times when you felt competent and confident, and again choose the best one."

Abigail: "As I think about it, I felt secure whenever I spent the night at my grandparents' house on weekends. My grandmother would tuck me into the big bed she had in the guest bedroom, and sing to me until I went to sleep. The sheets were really white and smelled so nice. I can almost hear her voice and the song she sang."

"Picture that scene in the guest room clearly. Be there in your imagination. See what you see, the shapes, the colors, the objects and furniture in that

room. Hear the sounds that you hear, noticing what you say to yourself at that moment of time. Now, pay attention to where you experience any sensations in your body. Memorize that feeling – and enjoy it thoroughly."

Abigail smiled broadly as she thoroughly remembered the details of that experience. The muscles around her eyes softened, and the wrinkles in her forehead smoothed out. She reported that she felt security, relaxation, and peace as well as breathing more easily, as she looked at that scene in her mind's eye.

The time when she felt the most confident and competent was when she had been given special recognition by her boss, a cash bonus, and a promotion when she sealed a lucrative contract with a client company. It was a wonderful kudo, a feather in her cap. The sensations she experienced when she thought about being confident were right in the center of her chest. She described them as being very warm, and large. When asked to recall what she said to herself, Abigail smiled broadly, made a fist, and exclaimed, **"I did it! Yay!"**

"Now, at one of those moments of anxiety with your boss, step into those resourceful feelings and imagine how having those feeling of security and confidence impacts and changes your feelings."

Abigail: "He was just being particular in how he wanted those reports. As I think of it now, he may have been concerned about criticism from

> *his boss. When I received that promotion, it was because I wrote a really good contract proposal, so he knows my writing skills are good. My worst fears were getting the best of me. That still should have had nothing to do with eating sweets."*

Abigail reported that she certainly has experienced other moments of anxiety, and her life is still not immune to frustrations, but she no longer eats sweets as a response to them.

Limiting Internal Beliefs

Some people develop and maintain such limiting, internal beliefs that they generate doubt about their very right to exist; much less to have the appearance that they want, or to enjoy being happy. A vicious cycle begins if you eat high calorie "comfort foods" to attempt to feel better. Inevitably, this will be followed by an experience of regret, guilt, and depression because the consequences of eating those foods affect the way your clothes fit. The cycle is complete if you blame the bad feelings on how much you weigh, and become discouraged as you think of your years of effort with few of the results that you wanted. Helplessness and hopelessness are created which become overriding existential beliefs. This generates the need to eat even more to get that temporary emotional comfort. And so the cycle continues and widens.

An empowering belief that includes competence, courage, and determination is the antidote. You can build this belief when you access those internal experiences from your past which embody evidence that you have the capacity to generate those resources.

Metabolic Set Point

Going through a plateau in what you weigh is the normal and natural way your body readjusts to a new weight and resets the metabolic 'set point'. Otherwise, your body may send signals to your brain to create a mind-set of 'starvation'. This give rise to more intense urges to eat quantities of those more familiar, high calorie foods. **Plan** to establish a plateau. Once it becomes a conscious choice, you continue to remain in control of the process.

> *Carol provided a wonderful example of how she used this strategy. She decided to maintain a stricter regimen for three weeks. Then, except for portion control, she took a 'vacation' from the restrictions for a one-week period and repeated this pattern for the duration of her action plan.*

Of course, you can decide for yourself to extend time you engage in a more disciplined practice and focus. This will certainly keep you energized to remain committed. When you notice that the needle of the scale seems stuck at a certain point, even though you have been faithful to your diet plan, it is important to recognize that it is a plateau and give yourself a break. In the same way that you find you are more energized and enthusiastic about getting back into the swing of things when you return to work after a vacation, you will find yourself even more committed after just a week-long hiatus. Your body will begin to re-start the calorie reduction. It is like three steps forward and one step backwards. You may be more gradual and lengthy in making progress, but on the other hand, it may be a little more palatable which helps increase persistence and commitment. As Mary Poppins sings, *"A spoonful of sugar makes the medicine go down."* That song is relevant and appropriate in this context. The winning is always long-term, and is a process rather than a race. This strategy will keep you energized and committed rather than discouraged. When you have started the ball rolling to get rid of even five to ten pounds of excess weight, your enthusiasm and determination will increase. You will actually see how your clothes fit differently on your body. Your energy level will increase as you get into the habit of working out regularly. Even more important, your self-esteem will improve as you continue to feel proud of your ongoing accomplishment.

Negative expectations, impatience, and discouraging self-talk can generate a low frustration tolerance, an imagined exaggeration of problems and their possible impact, as well as sadness or anger. All of these are self-defeating, and require more effective solutions than eating.

The antidotes to these limiting and undermining beliefs are simple to understand; and more complicated to accomplish, or in more common language: "easier said than done." Understanding that no one or nothing is perfect is a prerequisite to transforming these limiting beliefs. In fact, it's a wonderful permission to give yourself to accept and welcome your own vulnerability and faults; in short, your own **humanity.** Sure, you will be really successful and proud of yourself one day, and then really blow it the next. You have all been there! There will be imperfect people in your life; some of whom energize you, and some who deplete your energy. That is the purpose of being discriminating and selective about those with whom you socialize and connect.

Unconditional Self-Love

Accepting and loving yourself unconditionally, with all your flaws, is an important factor in winning your weight war. Does this mean that you should just accept your weight as is, and give up your personal struggle to get to your goal weight? Absolutely not! What it does mean is that you need to be a cheerleader for your ambitions and goals rather than being a critic.

Louise:

A talented, professional musician, Louise is thirty-nine years old, and has been married to her childhood sweetheart for twenty years. She has been struggling with weight all of her teen and adult life. She identified her present overeating as a response to being upset and frustrated by others at work and at home who view the world very differently than she does. Whenever she was criticized by a colleague or her husband, she felt disrespected, alienated, and unfairly treated. She kept a log of her objective observations about what actually happened just before she was emotionally upset. She then wrote down all of the internal dialogue or self-talk, which allowed her to interpret this objective reality. Louise could then identify her negative internal belief that since others evaluated and judged her poorly, she must not be acceptable. She worried that her performance was never good enough, even though she received many compliments. When asked for evidence of the truth of this awareness, Louise identified the constant criticism that she had received from her parents and older brother when she was young. The other limiting belief that is relevant to her weight was her own judgment that she was unattractive based on the taunting of her brother and his friends who made fun of her hair, her shyness, and of course, her weight.

To change this belief of inadequacy and get back in control, Louise began to recognize that she was giving undue power to her older brother, and even strangers, to determine whether or not she was nice, competent, or attractive. That put them on a power pedestal, which they **certainly** *did not deserve. Since she had assumed that her parents would have stopped the teasing if they had disagreed with her brother, the belief had been affirmed. In fact, after asking, Louise discovered that her parents had no idea of the emotional abuse that the brother had imposed on her, and therefore were unable to challenge it at the time. Since they had criticized her on other issues they thought were important, it felt as if everyone were 'piling on'. She then recognized how irrelevant this was to her present life by imagining how, as a child, she could adopt an adult perspective which could recognize her parents' personal limitations. (Her father was a hard-working immigrant, and her mother was submissive, and overwhelmed with the responsibilities of bringing up three children without much money. Neither was well educated.) Both wanted their children to succeed and so pressured them to achieve academic and financial success. After analyzing this history objectively, Louise adopted a verbal mantra every time she felt vulnerable and inadequate. Instead of eating, she would take a deep breath, let it all out and think;* **"I am a competent adult who is in control of making my destiny real! I can decide to make healthy** *food choices and eat only small portions." Louise was amazed that it was now easy to reject the earlier assumptions that she had made. She accepted her own values, ethics and integrity as the sole authority on which to base her self-esteem. Two months later, Louise was well on her way to winning her weight war.*

Resolving Personal Sabotages

It is very important to discover all the ways that you might sabotage your goal. What are the temptations that at any one moment seem more important to you than sticking to your commitment to win the war on your overweight? Make a list of those specific temptations to prepare your defenses to resist them. Is there a common element to the foods that are more tempting than others? Do they tend to be sweet, salty or crunchy? Is there a specific time frame that triggers those temptations? For example, are you inclined to be more tempted at night or in the middle of the afternoon? Are you more tempted when you are alone or with others? These temptations are tied up with the psychological needs that drive your overeating behaviors.

To feel strong in resisting temptations, it is important to 'program' your personal sense of competence and confidence into your unconscious awareness to recognize what it feels like to achieve goals that you have set. These are the resources that you need to feel confident about resisting temptation.

Past Successful Decision Strategy

How do you know when you are successful at meeting a challenge? If you think of past challenges in your life that you have had to overcome to achieve your goals, you can take courage and confidence in knowing that you have all the inner resources you need to achieve what you want.

When you examine and evaluate your past successful tactics for making decisions, you can utilize that positive model to influence your decisions about eating healthy food. Creating a reference experience of success is the key to your confidence in achieving goals that you set. That plan of action is the behavioral factor of success.

Creating a reference experience of success is the key to your confidence in achieving goals that you set. That plan of action is the behavioral factor of success.

> *Bob recounted the story of how he had quit smoking cigarettes after nearly fifteen years of smoking well over a pack a day. The turning point was having watched his mother decline in health while fighting lung cancer for almost two years. His mother spent long periods of time in the hospital hooked up to IV's and oxygen. Bob was determined that he would never put himself or his family through that torture. He had a hard time dealing with the resentment he felt for his mother, believing this was an illness that his mother imposed on herself by smoking. Every time he wanted a cigarette, or saw his co-workers or friends lighting up, he had reminded himself of the image of his mother dying in the hospital. Bob recalled that he had struggled with the temptation, particularly when*

he saw others light up and inhale. Since he had made up his mind to protect his health, he threw away his cigarettes. Bob remembered how he had gritted his teeth, and turned away from the smokers to concentrate on that powerful image of her mother in the hospital. It was more of a contest than he thought it would be – but he had won. Bob regarded this exercise as the 'skeleton key' to unlocking the doors that had kept his goal hidden. He was surprised that he had not put that resource to use before.

"What are the sensations that you experience when you are in touch with that sense of determination?"

Bob: "It was like a solid, centered, comfortable intensity in the chest. I also felt very proud of myself every time I said "no" to a cigarette."

"That's neat! Now be present in that moment of determination with that 'solid, centered, comfortable intensity,' and this time, focus on what you say to yourself at that moment in time."

Bob: "Hmm, I guess I am saying "I won't do that to myself. It's not worth it."

"Does your solid comfortable sensation increase or decrease when you say those words to yourself?"

Bob: "Oh, it definitely increases that determination".

"Super! Now, as you imagine being tempted to eat those cookies or potato chips which will put weight on, say to yourself, 'No I won't do that to

myself. It's not worth it!' and discover how you re-spond this time."

Bob: (After a long pause) "That's interesting; the cookies not only look less tempting, but I feel almost disgusted that I would eat something that would add to my weight. ... That's very different!"

Transforming Limiting Beliefs

Early in everyone's life, a belief begins to develop about the world and one's place or role in it. Beliefs are generalizations about the world which create emotional boundaries and "filters". These in turn, interpret reality in ways that either limit or empower you. They influence your ambitions and the choices you make: "Is the world a safe place in which to live? Can I trust the people with whom I live or have connections? Am I smart enough, good enough, worthwhile enough to dream—and achieve my dreams?" If these beliefs make your specific goals easier to achieve, then they are empowering. When they negatively impact your life and diminish your capacity to accomplish what you want, they become beliefs which limit your options, and need to be changed to allow you to achieve your goals. Robert Dilts, one of the foremost authorities on NLP, has written several wonderful books on how beliefs affect your health. The following is an adaptation of the "Reimprinting" strategy as explained in the book, *Beliefs: Pathways to Health and Well-Being,* which he wrote with Tim Hallbom and Suzi Smith.

Limiting beliefs are born as a child attempts to understand and interpret the intentions of adults when those caretakers or role models are critical, angry, upset, or even drunk. Because no young child has the wisdom or logic to interpret the events rationally, any interpretation is flawed. Decisions about whether or not that younger self is worthwhile or valued by important adults are made from these flawed interpretations. Since adults seem larger than life and magical to a young child, the conclusion is that child, herself, must be defective and wrong. The child then reverts to the only comfort she can count on and has any appropriate control over: eating food!

Experiencing resources

Now that you are an adult with wisdom, logic, and experience; you can be curious to discover what kinds of different emotional resources you would have needed in your early childhood to change those negative self-evaluations.

→ Recall events in your adult life when you have experienced those resources.

→ Imagine how you might have grown up differently if those resources had been part of your life then.

→ What do you need to believe that would have been be more empowering?

→ If needed, you can continue to create additional appropriate resources, or you can make those resources you already have, more intense or stronger until you feel comfortable.

→ Now imagine what your new belief would sound like, and what your new behavior would be in response to that recently created, empowering belief.

Lorraine recounted that she was brought up in a single-parent home as an only child. Her mother had often been moody and would yell at very minor errors or missteps. The only effective mechanism that Lorraine discovered would work well was to ask her mother for a sweet snack. When her mother would take the time to sit down to eat it with her, she mellowed out, and little Lorraine did not have to be so scared. This strategy had generalized as the primary means of calming herself down as an adult. She ate sweets from that point on — to calm her nerves, and to feel more in control. Intellectually, Lorraine knew that her mother did not engage in this behavior to purposely make her fat, but she also realized that she could not shift this negative behavior as long as she associated sweets with being safe. The belief that sweet food "calmed the threatening beast" when she was unable to fix it had become an 'imprint' experience because it continued to impact her behavior even though it was no longer appropriate.

Lorraine was told to identify the inner resources she now possessed as an adult that she could have used during that traumatic time. **Thinking logically** *was one of them. As she retrieved her favorite experiences of being logical, Lorraine felt centered and in control. Lorraine thought that her six-year-old younger self could have used an* **adult understanding and appreciation** *of just how worried and upset her mother must have been as she struggled to know how to support herself and her daughter.* **A sense of humor** *would have given that younger Lorraine a very different perspective on how her mother's moods and* *needs were different from hers. With that sense of humor, Lorraine imagined that she could create a situation comedy about her mother's behavior and attitude - similar to the comic genius of Roseanne Barr. The last resource that Lorraine thought that could have helped her younger self was **assertiveness** that she used in her present life to successfully ask for what she wanted.*

*Lorraine focused on incorporating and integrating all those resources into her image of that six-year-old person she had been so long ago. Then she replayed that scene to discover what had changed. She reported that she could now relate to her mother differently, and released herself from all responsibility for her mother's happiness. She gave **that** back to her mother. Not only was Lorraine able to see herself as a competent, conscientious woman who could make appropriate decisions, she took control of what she ate, how much she ate, and when she ate it.*

Summary:

Temptations are fueled by negative experiences, thoughts and beliefs about yourself and how you fit into life events. When you have a low frustration tolerance or are easily discouraged, you tend to revert back to old habits which represent security and comfort. The antidotes are to find more effective resources, whether from inside yourself or dependent on others, to satisfy those emotional and psychological needs. Reimprinting old limiting beliefs empowers you to adopt a winning mindset which gives a different understanding and appreciation of what had been assumptions since childhood.

In addition to eating small portions of healthy foods, you are fighting these battles with one hand tied behind your back if you are not burning off more calories and fat than it takes in. The following chapter concentrates on how **you** can turn your body into a fat-burning machine. Exercise is the key.

CHAPTER 9

Strategy Eight: Exercise Your Right to Be Slender and Fit (with Kip Jawish)

"Everyone nags and insists on exercise. If I diet, and reduce my intake of food, why isn't that enough?"

Our bodies are like complex machines. Their efficiency and effectiveness depends on the quality of the fuel that we use and the intensity and the frequency with which we put these "machines" into action to energize and fortify their entire systems. But the fact is that as complex as our bodies are, the way to win the weight war is surprisingly simple.

1. Fuel properly by eating high quality nutritious foods in appropriate quantities

2. Move more intensely to burn excess calories and fat, and to strengthen the cardio-vascular system

3. Start a strength building program to build lean muscle and increase the metabolism, which will help burn more calories twenty-four hours a day.

But if it is so easy, then why is obesity so prevalent? Sixty-five percent of Americans are overweight, including more than thirty percent who are considered clinically obese. Obesity not only doubles the mortality rate, and reduces life expectancy by ten to twenty years, but it also reduces the quality of life as well. So, what can be done when we **continually** win small battles (drop fifteen pounds on a fad diet) and then lose the war (gain twenty pounds back)?

The development of labor-saving devices and high technology has reduced the exercise we used to get by just doing regular housekeeping or home maintenance chores. The basic physical activity needs of our bodies have remained constant over the years. Stress is a physiological response of our bodies. While stress generates tension, shortness of breath, and constricted circulation, it also slows metabolism and inhibits digestion. Physical activity helps to lengthen muscle fibers, improves circulation and breathing, as well as activates stress-relieving hormones and speeds up the metabolic rate to help get rid of calories faster and more efficiently. Physically fit individuals report fewer health problems and more resilience when confronted with major life changes.

Metabolism and Exercise

So what is metabolism – and how do you increase it? Your metabolism is the sum of all chemical reactions in your body's cells that converts the food you eat into energy needed by your bodies for everyday activities from sleeping, to running, and everything in between. The more that you move, (and the more concentrated the movement) the higher your metabolism becomes, and you will burn off more excess calories and add lean muscle mass on your body. By adding just five pounds of lean muscle, you will burn almost an extra eight pounds of pure fat each and every year without any exercise whatsoever, for the rest of your life. By adding in aerobic exercise, you will stoke your metabolism even higher, and burn more fat in your body's metabolic furnace. Walking at 3.5 mph burns from 5.6 to 7 calories per minute. If you walked for one hour per day that would add up to almost another 45 pounds of fat burned per year! Imagine that. Just by walking one hour a day and lifting weights for one year, you will reduce your weight by more than fifty pounds. And that is without even making any changes to your diet. FIFTY POUNDS! See how easy it can be when you make exercise a habit.

Julie:

Julie came to us after her doctor recommended our studio to her to help her get to her goal weight, and be fit and healthy. She weighed 230 pounds on the first day I met her. Her energy was low, she had a grayish pallor, and her self-esteem was at rock bottom. After her first exercise sessions, she began to notice a difference in her energy level. She still wasn't 100 percent committed, but she felt better every time she left the studio. While it was still a struggle for her to come in, Julie claimed that knowing her personal trainer was waiting for her was a big motivation to show up three times a week. It was also important to her that she was investing her own funds to benefit from our help and expertise. We offered daily encouragement, positive reinforcement and a variety of exercises to keep her exercise sessions fun. At the end of her first month, Julie was actually looking forward to coming in. She told us that she didn't realize how poorly she had felt prior to beginning her exercise program. After she started working out, she could see the good effects of becoming healthy inside and out. Her skin was glowing, and her whole attitude had changed. Julie even hired a nutritionist to give her detailed nutritional guidance on healthy eating habits and meal planning. After six months, Julie had reduced her excess weight by 43 pounds, and gained six pounds of metabolically active lean muscle mass. Best of all, she moves, feels and acts like "a million bucks!"

Form an Exercise Plan

The initial step is to make a plan. To win the war you must attack the enemy from all sides:

1. Set obtainable, measurable goals

2. Design a healthy eating plan

3. Train both the muscles and cardiovascular system

4. Stay motivated so that your new plan becomes a habit, and remains a permanent part of your new healthy lifestyle

If I (Kip) could package all of the benefits of exercise and put them into a pill, I would be a millionaire tomorrow. But exercise and its benefits are free, and are as easy as putting on your sneakers and going for a nice long walk around the neighborhood. You need to make exercise a healthy habit.

How often, how long, where, when, what, with whom? These are questions you can ask yourself to keep yourself committed to the process of fitness and health. In addition to regular physical fitness workouts or weight-lifting, there are many other options that will help you get exercise in fun and unexpected ways:

→ Running and/or jogging (for the less intense enthusiasts) have been favorite options as witnessed by the large increase in the number of annual marathons in the U.S. and across the world.

→ Swimming is not only an inexpensive and fun way of exercising, but it is also a necessary ability and competence that could save your life when you are around water. It is a great form of exercise especially for obese people because of the buoyancy of the water. Someone who weighs over two hundred pounds can feel almost weightless in the water. With the popularity of indoor pools, swimming has become a true all-season activity. Swimming for exercise is different than jumping into the ocean, getting your hair wet, jumping waves and paddling around. As in all the strategies that you have been discussing, you will want to specify an achievable goal for yourself such as swimming hard for fifteen minutes, swimming ten laps, or perhaps, swimming the front crawl for ten minutes and the backstroke for an equal time. You are only limited by your energy and creativity. Make it fun rather than a chore!

→ Do you remember how you loved playing in the snow as a child? Using that wonderful wooden Flexible Flyer sled to figuratively fly down the big hill? Make winters fun for your children as well! If you have a sled, toboggan, or snow tube, or two, walk up the big hill with them and slide down again, at least ten times.

→ Snowboarding rivals skiing in popularity and both can be excellent and fun forms of exercise.

→ Invest in a pair of snow shoes or cross country skis, and explore the woods around you after it has snowed, while your neighbors suffer from cabin fever.

If you need a break at work, walk outside on nice days. On rainy, snowy, or cold days, walk inside around the halls. Make elevators your enemy – walk up and down the stairs. Park the car in the most distant space – so you can be energized when you sit down at your desk.

Most of us enjoy competitive team sports: watching from the stands or seated on our comfortable sofa or recliner, watching television, while *others* actually play the sports. Very few of us engage in playing ourselves, mostly because we tell ourselves that there are relatively few opportunities.

Exercise Options

Life isn't a spectator sport. You need to jump up off of your couch, and get into the game of living. All the following activities have informal teams, leagues, or pick-up games.

- ↪ Soccer

- ↪ Softball

- ↪ Baseball

- ↪ Hockey

- ↪ Basketball

- ↪ Badminton and volleyball are sports that you can enjoy playing, even with a relatively small number of people.

- ↪ There has even been a revival in the appeal of the old schoolyard games of kickball and dodgeball.

Engage in a familiar activity that may or may not be competitive and which will burn calories while you are having fun. Learn some new active sports you can enjoy. Even less strenuous sports are better than sitting on your rear end.

- ↪ Tennis is a fun, social activity that can fit into a specific time frame.

- ↪ Bicycling

- ↪ Rowing

- ↪ Ice skating or roller blading

→ Skateboarding

→ Bowling leagues and teams are flourishing.

→ If you play golf, walk. If you don't walk, riding in a cart and playing golf is better than doing nothing.

Walking as Exercise

Let's discuss walking as exercise. It is without doubt one of the favorite non-organized ways of getting physical. Since most everyone has skill in walking, and there is a very low risk of injury, it is a wonderful way to build up your cardiovascular system and kick-start your fitness program. One wonderful advantage of walking is that, as exercise plans go, it is very inexpensive. The only requirement is a pair of quality running or walking shoes. Make sure they are comfortable, and designed for walking. They don't have to be expensive, but they do have to fit well. When you decide to walk, make it a regular appointment at the same time of day. Walk briskly with purpose. After a while, you can wear a weight vest and make the walking if you want to increase the amount of exercise that you get. You can choose a hilly course once or twice a week to challenge yourself. If you live in a flat landscape like the beach, you can take the steps rather than use an elevator. It will generate energy, improve your mood and enthusiasm, relieve tension, as well as burn up fat calories. You win by feeling proud of yourself for engaging in such a worthwhile activity.

Many indoor malls have measured the "distance" around the mall for walking, and may even open early in the morning so you can walk briskly to exercise, have plenty of parking, and can window-shop in the bargain.

It is important to dress appropriately for the weather. In the winter you should wear layers of clothes and a wind-breaker so you can be ready for any outside condition. Modern fabrics are designed to breathe, and wick excess heat and moisture away from the body. A hat that covers your ears and the top of your head keeps the majority of your body heat from escaping. Drink plenty of water to replace the body fluids that escape when you walk. Start slowly and build up your energy. If you walk outside, vary your route so it stays interesting. A walking buddy will keep you so engaged that the time and miles will seem like nothing.

Dancing

The TV show, *Dancing with the Stars* has inspired many people to consider dancing not only as a way to meet nice people, but also as a great way to exercise. Learn to dance – or **go** dancing if you already know how. You get to hear great music. It gets you off your rear – and onto your feet, moving your body to the beat, and having fun. Some types of dancing do not even require partners. It really doesn't matter if you choose to dance to country and western, pop-rock, polkas, waltzes, or the oldies-but-goodies. It *will* count as exercise. Square dancing and folk dancing will certainly help you burn off calories and count as aerobic activity. 'Aerobic Dancing' is a great way to listen to your favorite music and burn off calories at the same time.

There are many aerobic dancing and exercise tapes professionally made with music and physical fitness gurus (or wanna-be's) to demonstrate the steps, maintain the pace, make sure you stretch appropriately, and help you keep focused on how to move.

Mind-Body Connection

"Mens sana in corpore sano" means "Sound mind in a sound body". This Latin phrase is well known to many, but what does it really mean? The Romans knew that a healthy body was integral to keeping a healthy mind, and the Romans didn't need hundreds of studies or years of research to discover this correlation. This fact, however, has been lost in our modern world where prescription drugs have been the treatment of choice for most maladies of modern living. In any given one-year period over twenty million Americans suffer from depression, which is almost ten percent of the population. When new clients come into the fitness studio, they fill out a medical questionnaire. It is always surprising at how many are affected by depression, and are medicated as part of their treatment. After almost twenty years in the personal training profession, it still feels good when a client relates how much exercise has helped him or her with depression. It is a fact that a well-designed exercise plan, along with a specific nutrition program builds a strong foundation in the battle to combat the epidemic of obesity in our culture. The positive effects of exercise on physical well-being are well-documented, and these effects include changing the course of such illnesses as osteoporosis, hypertension, coronary heart disease, and cancer, as well as improving a sense of psychological well-being.

> **Cynthia:**
>
> *About ten years ago Cynthia came into the In-Fit studio, and we went over her fitness goals. She was a typical suburban housewife who wanted to drop about twenty pounds and to tone up her muscles. Almost immediately after her first workout, Cynthia's mental attitude noticeably improved. She started to gain self-confidence and felt better about herself with each workout. Months later, Cynthia confided to me*

that she had been taking medication for depression. She no longer cried herself to sleep at night since she had started exercising. She reported feeling mentally stronger as her physical well-being improved. To this day, Cynthia is still in fitness training three days a week. She has accomplished her goals through her exercise program, and her depression is kept under control, with lowered levels of her medication.

Exercise and enthusiasm

Almost on a daily basis, I hear stories about how exercise has helped to improve a client's emotional attitude as well as reducing their clothing size. Perhaps the most interesting shift that I have seen is the beneficial effect on family members who watch their significant others adopt a positive energy level and renew their enthusiasm.

Bob and Mary:

A couple named Bob and Mary contracted to have supervised workouts at their home. I had worked with Mary by herself for several weeks, until she convinced her husband that he should join her. He was a very successful businessman who owned several companies. A hard-driving man, he was very competitive in all aspects of his life - from the business world to the tennis court and golf course. He was under constant stress, and had the reputation of being quite a bear. (That was putting it mildly!) One day Mary pulled me aside and mentioned that since Bob had started working out, his blood pressure had lowered, and the quality of his sleep at night was enhanced as his snoring diminished. His moods had improved substantially; a fact that was noticed by many in his business and personal life. In short, he was a lot more enjoyable to be around. (Mary added, in passing, that he had reduced his weight by twenty pounds!)

If you are intimidated by big, sweaty gyms, you can turn your home into your own private personal training "studio" for very little money. All you need is a few dumbbells, a stability ball and an aerobic bench. You can do almost every exercise in the privacy of your own home that they have in large, impersonal fitness clubs. You may want to hire a certified, personal trainer to come into your home, and design a few personalized workouts for you to get you started. You can arrange for that trainer to regularly come by to teach you new exercises or create challenging modifications to the old ones that will keep your motivation and interest high.

Personal Trainer Benefits

That is why hiring a personal trainer can be so beneficial. They will measure your body fat, assess your fitness levels, and then gauge your progress over the course of your program. Your own personal trainer is an important resource to explain the value and purpose of each exercise he or she asks you to do. This helps you get on the motivational bandwagon to generate enthusiasm and excitement for making progress in getting fit. They can design a safe and effective exercise program, specific to your fitness goals and needs, as well as make appropriate adjustments as you progress. A good personal trainer will provide you with an environment to keep you on track with a maintenance program. There are many people who call themselves personal trainers, so you need to be careful. Make sure they are certified by a reputable organization. All of your trainers should be certified by the National Association of Sports Medicine (www.NASM.org). Ask for references and check them out. Also, ask for a free workout to see if you like the facility, the trainer, their personality, and training methods. You have a lot of choices, and you want to make sure your experience is a positive one. Committing yourself to personal fitness is indeed a lifestyle decision which can benefit you for years to come. Choosing an effective personal trainer and "fitness coach" will offer you a valuable ally to assist in designing a program to enhance your goals and values.

What if you can't afford a personal trainer? How can you stay motivated and consistent in your exercise to help you win your war on excess weight?

S.M.A.R.T. Goals

First, you need to write down your goals. What do you want to accomplish in two weeks? One month? Three months? Twelve months? Your goals need to be **S**pecific, **M**easurable, **A**ttainable, **R**ealistic and **T**ime-based or "**S.M.A.R.T.**"

> → **Specific**: such as "I want to get rid of ten pounds" instead of "I want to lose weight."
>
> → **Measurable**: setting a goal, such as dropping from 35 percent body fat to 25 percent.
>
> → **Attainable**: making a goal that is realistic, such as deciding to reduce ten pounds in one month, and then keeping it off. This is better than making a far-fetched goal which sounds great to start, but which will discourage you. A one to one-and-a-half-pound reduction in weight *per week* is considered healthy,

and more appropriate for achieving long-term weight reduction that lasts.

- **Realistic**: rejecting the thought of fitting into a size two when you have been a size twenty your whole adult life. A more realistic goal is to drop to a size fourteen, and then reevaluate your goals.

- **Time frame:** making some short term goals to keep you on track and focused towards your long-term goals. Also, post your goals where you can see them everyday and review them.

Most fitness studies state that the best way to reduce weight is not just to cut calories, to only lift weights, or to just do aerobics; but to *do all three* in an organized program designed to maximize both your efforts and results.

Jackie:

Jackie, a client of four years, said that since she lifts small weights, and does crunches while_she watches television, she does not feel guilty that she has wasted any time. She also hides the remote, so that when she wants to change the channels, she needs to move "just like in the olden days" before Tivo or remote gadgets. She organized an "exercise break" at work instead of one of the traditional coffee breaks, which was met with great enthusiasm from her co-workers.

Saboteurs

One thing you have to beware of is that not everyone wants to see you succeed. There are some people out there that would like nothing better than to see you fail for all kinds of reasons. They may be envious of your commitment to your good health, or they may want to relieve their own guilt for not being in control of their health by having you fail in your efforts. They may tempt you to have that greasy cheeseburger at lunch, or will keep bringing candy or donuts to your desk. These saboteurs may even schedule social events or business meetings which conflict with times that you regularly work out, so that you have to make a choice. Don't give in to them. Be strong, and keep telling yourself that you are *worth* the extra effort. These people may be family members, co-workers, or even your spouse. It may be your boss or your best friend, but just remember that you have a choice and that you are in control.

So what happens when friends and family try to sabotage your successes either knowingly or unknowingly? The best way to get them on your side is to let them know what your goals are, and how important achieving them has become for you. You can ask for their help and understanding, and suggest specific ways that each of them can contribute to your success. The rest is up to you. *It will not always be easy, but it is always worth it.* The **first** time that you turn down that donut at breakfast or those M&Ms at work is the hardest, and it will be *very* empowering. It becomes easier the more that you do it. Cravings become like waves on the ocean that you learn to ride out instead of drowning in them. If you don't succumb to the cravings, they will diminish. You can then replace them with something healthy and nourishing to your body. or just get out of your chair and walk around the hallways or the building until the temptation passes.

Summary:

Diseases of lifestyle are responsible for half of all deaths. Physical health, mental health and spiritual health can all be enhanced and improved through regular, consistent exercise. All of the benefits of a well-designed fitness program and a healthy lifestyle and philosophy are too numerous to mention. Some of the benefits that you can expect are reduced cardiovascular disease, lower blood pressure, lower cholesterol, less dependence on medication and lower risk of cancer to name just a few. For a commitment of just one hour a day with a slow steady change in unhealthy lifestyle habits you can reap all of the benefits of a new lifestyle that will not only add years to your life but will make those years the most enjoyable of you life. What are you waiting for—an invitation? Get off of the couch and start your active, new lifestyle now! You won't regret it!

The next chapter offers some effective strategies so you can maintain your sense of control and enjoyment when you go out to eat.

CHAPTER 10

Strategy Nine: Successful Restaurant Strategies

Eating in a restaurant is enjoyable. It provides a change of pace, a taste of foods from different cultures or foods that you might not otherwise prepare. Restaurants can provide an element of privacy for some who want time to recapture intimacy, an opportunity to reinforce good manners and appropriate public behavior for children, and a socializing opportunity for others to get together without work conversations or the responsibilities of shopping, cooking, and cleaning up afterwards.

On the other hand, for those who are battling their particular bulge, restaurant eating can be a daunting experience. How do you continue to be conscientious about what you choose to eat when you are not in control of how that food might be prepared or of the quantity of food you consume. Many people become overwhelmed by the number of choices, and the challenges of discriminating between them.

Marilyn

Marilyn frequented a restaurant near her home that served large portions with many starches and a variety of fried food. The only salad that was offered with any meal was Cole Slaw. The tossed green salads were only offered 'a la carte'. Marilyn noticed that the advertised choices in many of "fast food" chain restaurants are filled with calories and high carbohydrate choices such as French fries, fried chicken or double cheeseburgers with their famous sauces. These are loaded with saturated fat calories from frying which diminish the value of protein from the chicken or beef. This would not be the case if the food had been broiled or baked. Even potatoes have high nutrition value when they are baked, broiled, or steamed. She found that she could select restaurants which were happy to prepare their menu foods according to her requests. As she became a 'regular', they would even make suggestions about how they could customize some of their nightly specials to meet her dietary requirements. Fast food restaurants provide the advantages of low prices, convenience, and an informal atmosphere – not to mention efficiency of service. If you are careful and observant, you can discriminate between the high fat and high calorie options offered even at the fast food restaurants. These days, every fast food restaurant has healthy options. That is why "Subway" has been so successful in marketing "Jared" and his successful, low-fat diet choices. Check the calorie and fat content of food from any fast food chain on the Internet so you have all the information to make conscious and healthy decisions.

All You Can Eat Buffets

All-You-Can-Eat buffet options in restaurants are complex. This is both the good news **and** the bad news. There are many choices of food; some of uneven taste and quality. It's difficult to keep large quantities of food hot, cooked properly, and tasty. The real problem is that many people believe that they must eat great quantities of food in order to get their money's worth. The secret to enjoying buffets is to understand that you are paying for the **privilege of choice.** Taking small portions of different foods will provide samples of unique taste sensations. If some food doesn't measure up to your expectations; your calorie, taste or quality standards, ask either for a replacement order, or for your money to be refunded. Another option is to just leave it on the plate.

You can play a psychological game to fool the eye (trompe d'oeil) if you are used to seeing full plates of food. Use smaller dessert-size plates to help you feel satisfied and comfortable with small portions. Remember that you can have small portions, and taste little bits of many foods, or you can choose just a few foods that you really like. Keep in mind that you will want to be cautious about consuming large quantities of high calorie foods. You can often look at restaurant web sites ahead of time, so you can make logical decisions, and plan your meals in advance.

The following strategies will provide you with an empowering mindset to be in control of decisions about what you eat - and what you weigh.

Successful Strategies

When you look at a menu in a restaurant, take the time to thoroughly check it out in terms of the types of food offered, whether or not it will help you or prevent you from reaching your weight goals, and pick out a few things that instinctively appeal to you. Make a picture of what each of them might look like, and imagine what each might taste like. Ask yourself – *"Is this worth the cost in terms of the possible **taste value, health value, or price value** as well as the **number of calories** in each of those items?"*

Remember to include your future self in making menu or buffet choices in a restaurant. She is the essence of all the benefits that you will have as a result of getting to your goal weight. Decide on what choices you can reject as NOT being worth the calories? Go through a similar decision-making process with each possibility. It's important to think about what foods you will want to choose to reject in the future, if what you select is very tempting and full of calories. If you chose something with fewer calories on the menu now, and eat a sensible quantity, you might preserve your ability to choose a treat later.

If it is not possible or practical to take a 'doggie bag' or container of leftovers with you when you leave, remember: **"It is better to let 'leftovers' go to waste in a garbage can than to have them go to waste on *your waist*."**

Top 20 Restaurant Strategies

1. Research some specifics about your restaurant choices. Have you been there   before? Do friends recommend the food, the service, the menu?

2. Even though someone else might be picking out the restaurant, you are the only one who is in control of what **you** put in your mouth. For example if you are taken to a pizza parlor, you can order a cheese-less pizza, or grilled vegetables over the tomato sauce without the cheese. Many 'California' style pizzerias will feature very healthy or 'slimming' assortment of toppings.

3. Read through the menu completely from the appetizers to the beverages and desserts. This will allow you to get a complete sense of the available choices, and to properly evaluate how these options fit into your values and goals.

4. Think about the kinds of foods that you are in the mood to eat. Sometimes you might feel like seafood, other times you could be more in the mood for a Caesar salad, Italian food etc.

5. Eliminate from consideration those foods that do not fit your mood.

6. Check with the image of your 'future self' as your ally to determine if that choice will help you win this battle, or whether or not it could keep you from it. If none of the menu options would satisfy both your taste buds, your value system and your stated goals, you have the alternative of leaving the restaurant, changing your mind about what you want to eat, or looking for ways of modifying the choices to better fit your specifications.

7. Reduce the food choices to only those which will fit all of those criteria.

8. Make a colorful image in your mind's eye of how that choice might be prepared and what it might look like. Imagine what it will taste like if it is fixed that way. If you don't have enough information to make a thorough visual representation of that choice, ask your server how it is prepared – then add **that** information to your decision-making process.

9. Investigate the calories and fat content of chain or fast-food restaurant entrees on-line.

10. Join with a 'partner' in your battle, so you can exercise together, go out to eat together and support each other.

11. Look forward so much to your entrée choice that the rolls, crackers, bread, or nacho chips will be less appealing, or ask that the server to remove those temptations from the table.

12. Order an appetizer as an entrée. The portions are smaller, the prices are lower and the taste is just as good.

13. Keep in mind that your stomach is just a little larger than your fist. Stop eating when you have eaten that quantity. There will **always** be more food to eat. Only eat until you feel **comfortable** rather than full.

14. **Eat very slowly**, so you can thoroughly enjoy the taste sensations of the food you have ordered, which the taste buds and saliva provide.

15. Desserts are the 'gravy' for the restaurants' cash flow. This is why the server either asks "Have you saved room for our wonderful desserts?" or "What would you like for dessert - our special cheesecake or a hot fudge sundae?" The other ploy that restaurants use is to bring out a tray full of those delicacies so that you can **see** the actual product rather than visualize it from a verbal or written description. If you find a dessert choice that ranks highest on your scale of desirability, plan your meal to account for those extra calories, and take your time as you eat it to enjoy it thoroughly without guilt. Be extra disciplined in your choices in the following days and weeks.

16. Plan on a "doggie bag" or a "take-out container" to take home what you do not finish. Use it for lunch or for dinner the next day.

17. Share an entrée, with perhaps a side salad for each.

18. Order from the Senior Menu, which provides smaller portions as well as a lower price.

19. Once again, if it's not possible to take anything back with you, let it go. Remember: "It is better to let 'leftovers' go to

waste in a garbage can than to have them go to waste on **your** waist."

20. Remember you can order the food to **your** specifications:

↪ Put any sauce or dressing on the side.

↪ Halve an order.

↪ Order food without salt, butter, or cream sauce.

↪ Ask for vegetables that may accompany other entrees.

↪ Entrees that are blackened may be ordered with the spices shaken on, which gives you all of the flavor with fewer calories.

Summary:

Remember, restaurants can be wonderful allies. Enjoy the advantages. You are sometimes more in control of what you eat than you are at home, when the kids are screaming for spaghetti, cheeseburgers, fries, or tacos, etc. Choose the kind of restaurant that will get you the biggest value for your money. Remember to include your future self in making your restaurant food choices. You are responsible for bringing her into reality. You can only do that by making healthy food choices. Preserve your logic and determination to eat responsibly and slowly. Stop when you have reached a "fist-fulfilling" quantity. Take the rest back with you in a "to-go" bag, or let the excess food go to waste in the garbage can rather than "going to waste on your waist!"

To focus on how you want to be in control of what you eat in your own kitchen, check out the next chapter. The suggestions are terrific, and you will find yourself closer and closer to victory.

CHAPTER 11

Strategy Ten: Win the Cooking Game with Jane Mercado, MA, LCPC

This chapter is about celebrating food. It will help you understand the significance of the nutritional considerations that your body requires and craves in the interest of maintaining your good health. You can learn winning strategies of preparing nutritious foods from easy-to-follow, delicious recipes, which limit fats and sugars to develop and maintain healthy eating habits. This is set up **so** well, you don't even miss the fats and sugars. You too can be an AVID cook and create and find wonderful dishes that are **healthy, as well as tasty**. These cooking ideas will be presented with accompanying recipes. Please know that this is not a "cook book", but rather a guide that can teach you some new approaches to preparing healthy food. Many of these options are not expensive, so they should fit easily into a normal food budget. This way you can use these suggestions to discover even more creative tactics for yourself, as you adapt your own favorite foods and recipes.

Tasty Strategies

To put it simply, change your techniques of food preparation and create new ways to enjoy the old favorites. The following are successful strategies that actually work, **and** are very tasty:

- ↪ Eat smaller meals more often throughout the day. (See Lunch Box.)

- ↪ Completely avoid the "white stuff": such as refined flour and sugars, et cetera, because they are "poisonous" to your weight outcomes as they increase appetite and cravings.

→ Drink at least eight glasses of water a day as it flushes out the toxins from the body.

→ Eat more fiber, less fat, and lots of fruits and vegetables.

→ Hire a trainer, and spend additional time at the gym.

→ Walk often and regularly.

Stopping any of the above would be retreating, and returning to the yo-yo way things used to be. This new life style works well. Perhaps the following suggestions and possibilities will give you a jump start that will help you win your "battle of the bulge."

Changing Negative Thoughts

At the risk of being repetitive, you have to change your thoughts and attitudes in order to change your behavior. It sounds easy and logical, but you probably know it's more complicated. For example, if you think that a healthy lifestyle is boring and unsatisfying, the chances of developing the necessary healthy eating strategies will be greatly reduced. On the other hand, you can transform any negative attitude into positive affirmations such as: *"Eating nutritious food and creating a healthy lifestyle can be fun and satisfying"*. This is a critical key to your success.

Another method to successfully changing negative thoughts takes only three steps:

1. Write down the negative attitude or thought.

2. Accept it as something that gets in your way. Own it, and be responsible for it.

3. Create a new, positive thought instead. *Rehearse it over and over* until it completely replaces the old unhealthy or unwanted thought.

Take the following statement for example: *"I don't have enough time in my busy day to take care of myself properly, by doing all the extra things that are required."* To rewrite that as a positive thought might sound something like the following: "I will **make** the time to be as healthy as I can be." The key word is **"MAKE"** the time. This may mean re-organizing your schedule, planning ahead, or putting your own needs before those of others. This might sound selfish at first glance, but the more you take care of yourself, the longer you will be able to effectively take care of others you love. Think about this with the same mindset that airlines use when they insist that you put on your own oxygen mask before helping those who are dependent on you. If we aren't healthy ourselves, it would be difficult to keep those around us healthy.

Take some time to think about your health habits, write them down and take a long hard look at your beliefs. Then re-write them as needed, and allow your 'internal cheerleader' to encourage you, and move you forward toward winning your battles.

Healthy Lifestyle Cooking Strategies

If you love to cook, and are willing to jump into this winning plan, you can learn how to prepare, cook and enjoy **real** food that is healthy and delicious. You will probably need to make some changes in your kitchen before you can get started. Remember, it takes time to change your lifestyle, especially if you have been responsible for cooking and feeding your family and friends.

There are so many new healthy brands on the market which are ahead of the game for you to try. You will certainly find your own favorites so that you can stop fighting with yourself, and you can enjoy the adventure of exploring the many winning possibilities available in local markets, and in your own kitchen.

Cleaning Out the Kitchen

Let's start by 'cleaning out' the kitchen. This idea is very different than keeping it clean! It is important to keep foods out of your kitchen that are useless to healthful nourishment.

Get rid of all the white flour, white sugar, white rice, white breads, pasta, unhealthy fats, fiber-less crackers, and especially the prepackaged mixes, or canned fruits stored in syrup. These staples need to be replaced with whole-grain healthier choices which taste just as good, if not better. Supermarkets have wonderful selections of high quality "healthy" foods. Of course, this requires that you spend time developing your own criteria of the food which will help you reach your goal. Time spent learning about basic nutrition facts as well will really help you in making wise decisions, which will become more automatic as you practice doing it. Spend the time necessary to read the labels *before* you buy food. It may seem hard and time consuming initially, but once you get the hang of it, it's as easy as A, B, C.

Tools That Really Help

Every battle needs the appropriate weapons. You will want to acquire the following culinary tools to help you win:

➥ A non-stick grill pan that fits over two burners on the stove. (This can be found in a good department store)

➥ A non-stick skillet

- A large strainer (not a colander)

- Small containers with lids for single portions

- Small "Ziplock" snack size bags (or equivalent)

- Ice cream scoop (1/2 Cup)

Basic Nutritional Information

It is important to have some basic nutritional information in order to shop appropriately and effectively. Evaluate the amount of sugars in food. It is generally agreed that Americans consume more sugar than any other food. This is because sugar is included in many of your prepared foods. Any ingredient that is labeled as containing either an *"ose"* or an *"ol"* suffix is made up of sugar. Fructose, sucrose, glucose, dextrose, lactose, or sorbitol are all good examples. All syrups have sugar calories at their base, whether they are made of corn, molasses, honey or maple. Most people who are overweight have a difficult time metabolizing sugars, since they are transformed into fat, and stored. You have probably heard that sugars are used by our bodies as fuel for energy because they break down easily. Our bodies use up the simple carbohydrates such as pasta, bread, or pretzels first. So far, so good! Finally, the body gets to burning off the complex carbohydrates such as vegetables, brown rice, or whole grains starches, etc. Since fat molecules seem to be the Ziplock storage bags for energy, the body tends to only burn off this fat *last*. When you reduce the amount of sugars from our bodies, you force your natural biological mechanisms to begin burning off the more complex carbohydrates, proteins and finally, fats.

Food changes your brain chemistry as it attempts to 'fill up' the emotional holes, literally as well as figuratively. You tend to relax or become energized, depending on what you put in your mouth. Emotionally, food may represent happy, positive experiences such as a celebration, reward, or success. Problems may arise when your activity levels go down below what is required to efficiently burn those calories off, so they are just pushed under the rug (or under the skin, so to speak) and stored as fat. As we saw in the last chapter, the whole idea of exercise is to efficiently burn off excess fat calories.

Shopping the 'New Way'

You will want to have **healthy** staples on hand. Flours, grains, breads, pastas, and crackers must be WHOLE GRAIN, which can be a mix of many grains, or just one grain if you prefer. The only caveat is that **whole *wheat*** products usually have only **one** gram of fiber as opposed to the ***three*** grams, or more that whole *grains* contain. This highlights the need to practice reading labels regularly to make healthy choices automatic. With such foods as boxed crackers, you will want to check the amount of fiber available, as well as the fat content. Fiber is a critical element in determining healthy choices. For a more detailed understanding of this important concept, see the 'Tips' section of this chapter. Make a habit of comparing the descriptions on the labels of different products. It takes more time at first, but as you discover the differences, you will know what you prefer. The organic food section usually offers more fiber choices with less fat.

When choosing beef or pork, select the leanest piece available. It may cost a little more, but remember the *cost* of defeat in your battle to win your war, if you don't spend the extra cash. Cut off all the visible fat before cooking, and absorb the liquefied fat with paper towels.

If you are cooking a whole chicken, make sure you take the skin off before eating it. All the fatty tissue is stored just under the skin. If you are using the skinless chicken breasts, use spices liberally, and cover it well, so the natural juices are kept inside. Using the recommended "grill pan" is a great way of cooking them.

Oat bran cereal boxes (Quaker Oats) have a muffin recipe that is both healthy and very tasty. TLC/Kashi creates wonderful cereal snack bars, chewy or crispy, usually found in the organic section. You can buy all kinds of ready-made fat-free or sugar free items which will be very helpful in creating great meals. "I Can't Believe It's Not Butter" spray, fat-free half-and-half, low fat cottage cheese, plain yogurt (with no sugar), many choices of dry cereal, skim milk (or 1 percent) if you prefer.

'Free' Foods

These are foods which are low in fats and carbohydrates. They are healthy, tasty, and will help you stay committed to eating well over your lifetime.

- Fresh fruits

- Canned fruit in fruit juices only

- Fruit frozen without sugar

- Fresh vegetables

- Vegetables frozen without sauces

- Egg substitutes or egg whites

- No-sugar Jell-O

Clearly, this is not a complete list by any means, but a beginning just to get you started. These are the foods that will not add to your weight as long as you **control the quantity** to no more than a "fist-full" to avoid stretching your stomach.

Use sugar substitutes as you wish. Always remember to portion out your servings for one portion. Make compromises for yourself, lowering the amounts of sugars and fats (healthy or not, they still have the same calories), increasing the amount of fiber, and avoiding the "white" stuff altogether.

What *Can* I Eat?

To win this war on overweight, it's important to focus on all the wonderful foods you **can** eat, rather than those which you want to limit or avoid. The purpose of this section is to look at some ideas for menus to prepare for dinners, and to use the leftovers for use in the "lunch box". The following healthy menu items are illustrative of the kinds of foods you can create. These are all delicious recipes that are used frequently.. There are many other possibilities either from low-fat cook-books, or your own family recipes for which you can use these examples as ways of adapting them. Recipes for starred items are included in the appendix.

1. *Fish and veggies in parchment or foil packs, baked in the oven.
2. Stir fry from bagged veggies and chicken. (Buy roasted chickens at the supermarket and remove the skin.)
3. *Pork tenderloin with dried fruit.
4. *Low-fat chili.
5. Soups (canned soups should be clear rather than creamy, or make your own)
6. *Fish with fruit salsa.
7. Flat bread homemade pizza.
8. *Frittata Florentine.

9. *Stuffed Portobello mushrooms.

10. *Grilled squash and eggplant with * marinara sauce.

11. *Lamb kabobs marinated in rosemary.

12. Flank steak.

13. *Roasted vegetables.

14. *Lasagna made with grilled vegetables instead of pasta.

15. *Spaghetti squash with your favorite Italian sauce.

Breakfast ideas would include:

1. Using eggbeaters and leftover vegetables to make an omelet.

2. Turkey bacon, Canadian bacon, or ham instead of regular bacon.

3. Smoothies.

4. Cooked or dry cereals with fruit and skim milk or fat-free half and half.

5. High protein breakfast bar and a banana.

6. Hard boiled egg (to grab and run).

7. Plain yogurt and low-fat granola and/or fresh or frozen fruit.

8. Home baked oat bran muffins (recipe on the oat bran box).

9. "Vita Muffins" sold in organic freezer section.

You will find that adapting these recipes and shopping for the basic food staples you need for healthy eating can be a fun challenge, almost like a game. With proper planning, the same foods that you prepare for dinner can be used for lunch or snacks by following the "lunch box" theory.

Lunch Box Theory

What do you think would happen if you could arrange to eat all day long and never feel hungry – without putting on a pound? Now what would you think if you could arrange to eat all day long, **and** make progress toward your goal weight? The "Lunch Box" theory is based on the idea that 'suffering is optional' in properly taking care of yourself.

"I don't have enough time to do that." How often have you said that to yourself or to others? Usually the first casualty of your time crunch is your health: exercise, vitamins, eating healthy foods, getting enough sleep, and really rewarding yourself on a daily basis for all your hard work and for all the good things you do. Taking the necessary time and energy to take care of your own health needs is important, but it often gets ignored in order to fully satisfy everyone else's needs.

What if **someone** in your life prepared a lovely lunch box of food that was healthy, well-balanced, and would **last** all day long? It would even contain the foods you need which have the number of calories that you need everyday. You could take this box with you, anywhere, and munch on it all day long whenever you wanted. This wonderful person took the time and effort to go to the grocery store and shop – **just** for you. She read the labels, found all the items in the right proportion to win your battles. Sometimes, as this favorite food was in a large bag or box, she would take it all back home, and put the food into small snack bags or containers to be put in *your lunch box.* If eating "three square meals" a day has resulted in your packing on more weight than is healthy for you, you deserve to experiment with eating many small meals a day. This doesn't mean that you can never have a feast or go out to dinner. This is all about protecting yourself from overeating or from eating foods that are not in your best interest, particularly at the end of the day, when you finally get a chance to relax.

"Lunch Box" Psychology

The fact is that **you** can be that caring person who will plan, shop, and fill the lunch box for you. Once you get started, it's very easy, and rapidly becomes a part of your weekly or twice-weekly trips to the grocery store. Remember to invest in a really nice, insulated lunch box, large enough to hold a "six-pack." Put two frozen water bottles in the bottom. It will serve two major purposes: the first is to keep the food cold and the second is to refresh you throughout the day. Make a drawer or a shelf in your refrigerator that is reserved just for you and your healthy food choices. Some clients have depended on their lunch boxes even when they were working from home, just because it was easy, handy, and there were no decisions to think about during the day.

You have the ultimate flexibility to adjust the items you put into your lunch box according to the events planned for the evening. For those of you who enjoy the game of counting calories to manage your weight, let's say that you want to limit your intake to twelve hundred calories a day. You can figure out the dinner calories you want to enjoy; and discover how much you have left to include in your lunch box for the rest of the day. Remember that vegetables are basically free to use with no worry about adding to your weight. Of course, this is dependent on remembering the "fist-full" image of the quantity of all foods that can satisfy your taste and nutrition needs.

Your lifestyle change does not mean 'all or nothing'. It is important to include fiber and complex carbohydrates in your meal planning. By choosing some sugar-free and some fat-free items, you will be able to enjoy many taste sensations and many different kinds of foods. When you find a label that reads, "No added sugar," with the fat content for each serving at three grams, it probably means that it would be a reasonable choice for a snack. This example is an attempt to get the thought process on track in evaluating what to select. The reading list on other books, resources, and articles will give you information to help you further analyze and evaluate your choices. Once you have the information, you can develop your own shopping guidelines with thought and mindfulness. You will always be experimenting and compromising, which is the essence of being in control of what you weigh. Remember that your progress toward your goal needs to be healthy, consistent, and satisfying as opposed to drastic and rapid.

Some possibilities to include in your lunch box are listed below. All of these have been personally taste-tested with the "Jane Mercado Seal of Approval."

- Puddings (no sugar or no fat)

- No-sugar Jell-O

- Fruit and Jell-O combination cups

- Small containers of cottage cheese

- Healthy snack bars (Try TLC/Kashi in the organic sections)

- Applesauce, no sugar (in the small cups)

- Low-fat graham crackers

- V-8 Juice

- Low-fat cheese sticks

The above items are all prepackaged. Some great "combo" ideas follow. Eat your applesauce with one serving of low-fat graham crackers. (It is reminiscent of apple pie.) Enjoy a piece of fruit with your cheese stick. There are many others that you can create.

The following are some additional ideas of enhancing your daily lunch box choices. Some of these will require some organizing and pre-packaging into smaller quantities.

➥ Dijonnaise spread is a no-fat cross between Dijon mustard and mayonnaise, and is found in the mustard section.

➥ Frozen pre-cut grilled chicken breast slices.

➥ Low-fat ham or turkey.

➥ Try turkey pastrami or bacon (very low fat).

➥ Alpine Lace Swiss Cheese (low-fat and thin sliced).

➥ Bagged salad.

➥ Hard-boiled or pickled eggs.

➥ Individual servings of Lite-Ranch dressing.

➥ Raw vegetables.

➥ No-sugar pickles.

➥ Fresh fruit cups or whole fruit.

➥ Marinated cooked vegetables in nonfat dressings (recipe to follow).

➥ Trail-mix in small amounts.

Making It Happen!

It's fun to explore new options and approaches to cooking and adapting *your* favorite recipes. The following cooking methods and recipe ideas can be adapted with all varieties of veggies and dressings of your own choosing. Notice that there is no oil or sugar in these recipes. In many cases, you will need to increase the taste and flavor level with additional herbs, onions, garlic, lemon and its zest (scrapings from the rind), pepper and a little salt to taste. Rice wine-vinegar can come in flavors or unflavored. You can control the sweetness, by selecting the unflavored vinegar. It is very light and very different from any other vinegar you may have tried. Make sure you taste as you go, so that you stay in control.

Marinated vegetables

Using leftover cooked vegetables which are drained and tossed in your favorite 'lite' or 'low-fat' salad dressing is a wonderful way to get your quota of vegetables every day. Keep them covered and refrigerated; they will last all week, and will certainly travel well. One cup is a serving. Try out the following yourself. You can experiment using your favorite vegetables or spices. More favorite recipes are included in Appendix X.

Fun with fruit – without wasting it

One of the problems with fresh fruit such as peaches, plums, pears, apples, or bananas is that it ripens quickly and begins to spoil. Grapes keep well in the refrigerator and freeze nicely for a cool, refreshing treat. When fruit is past its prime, my solution is to slice it up and bake it like a pie without the crust using Splenda and pie spices. Apples and bananas mix well, and of course you can freeze slices of ripe bananas in baggies to use in your healthy muffin recipes. You can even add them into smoothies.

You can create a lovely sauce when you heat ripened fruit in a saucepan with Splenda to taste, a pinch of salt and ¼ cup water for about 2 to 3 minutes after it comes to a boil. Choose your favorite fruit and the combinations. Some supermarkets sell bags of frozen mixed fruit without sugary additives, or you can use the frozen cut-up bananas you have stored. (See more recipes in Appendix X.)

Berries in the freezer

Put your choice of berries on a cookie sheet and freeze. Transfer them to sandwich-sized baggies for use on everything: cereal, yogurt, smoothies or anything else that stirs your imagination. You can buy them when they are in season and use them all year long.

Fruit salad or cocktail

Combine any 4 cups of your choice of cubed fruit combine well with ¼ cup lime or lemon juice and toss. You won't miss the sugary stuff at all, and it will keep much longer.

"Skinny Tomatoes"

The Italians use fresh tomatoes when they are in season. The rest of the year, they use the wonderful variety of canned tomato products, which have been picked and canned at the peak of the season, as well as tomato paste and sun-dried tomatoes. Even off-season Roma or grape tomatoes have great flavor if the recipe calls for fresh tomatoes. Tomato paste and dried tomatoes are sweeter and denser than other products, and give a different flavor to your dishes. The paste can come in a tube, which makes measuring out small amounts easier, faster, and you can keep it in the fridge efficiently. The two recipes below are useful to make ahead of time, and have them on hand in the refrigerator or the freezer. Of course, if you freeze the fresh sauce, the texture will change when you thaw it. The nutritional value will remain. It may be one of the many compromises we make in the name of efficiency.

Indoor Grilling:

With your non-stick grill pan, you can cook many delicious foods that are healthy, and that will help you win your weight war. The ridges keep the food away from the fat, and give it a nice flavor. An important point to note is that all non-stick pans should be warmed up slowly, and kept at a steady, medium heat rather than turning the burners on HIGH. Just give it several minutes. When you can't keep your hand three inches above the pan for more than a few seconds, you will know that the grill pan is ready. Below are some fun approaches in using your grill pan to create healthy recipes that will have your family and friends asking for more!

Eggplant and squash slices:

➥ **Slice the vegetables** about ¼ **inch** lengthwise

- **Brush lightly** with olive oil

- **Add salt and pepper** to taste

- **Place on grill** for 3-4 minutes undisturbed to allow grill marks to develop

- **Turn** for an additional 2 minutes

- **Serve** as a side dish or as part of a more complex recipe, instead of pasta.

  If you cook them too long, they will become soft and mushy. They can replace lasagna noodles, and you can layer them with your favorite sauces for casseroles. You also have the option of spraying the vegetables with Pam, adding pepper and salt, and broiling them. Make sure to watch them closely as they brown to turn them over before they burn. They are delicious in a casserole, sprinkled with Parmesan cheese, topped with tomato slices, and baked at 350 degrees until hot and bubbly (around 20-30 minutes).

Grilled Fruit

Peaches, plums, nectarines, or pineapple slices – Halved, sprayed with Pam. (If desired, you can dip fruit in Splenda before grilling.)

- Place the fruit on the grill **cut side down** for **4 minutes.**

- Serve grilled sides up.

- Use as a side dish, or with sugar-free toppings as a dessert.

Meat and Fish

Grilling meats give them a great flavor. If your cut is very thick such as pork tenderloin or a chicken breast, grill it on both sides until brown; then finish the cooking time for another 20 minutes in a 350 degree oven.

Grilling works well for thick fish steaks such as salmon or swordfish; whereas more delicate types of fish, like tilapia or flounder would do better when browned, and cooked in a non-stick skillet with Pam or 1 teaspoon olive oil.

Option two:

→ **Marinate the slices** of meat for 2 to 4 hours, (the thicker the cut, the longer the marinating time). Marinate fish for only 30 to 60 minutes and pat dry.

→ **Spray** with Pam or brush with olive oil

→ **Grill** until desired doneness.

Roasting Vegetables

This is another family favorite:

→ Using 6 of each: **carrots, parsnips or any other "root" veggie, and small redskin potatoes,**

→ **Preheat oven to 400 degrees.**

→ **Cut veggies to equal sizes** and arrange in a large roasting pan or cake sheet (1 to 2 inch pieces)

→ **Toss** with 1 tablespoon crushed **rosemary, garlic powder, pepper,** (optional) **salt,** and only enough **olive oil** to coat lightly (2 tablespoons or spray with Pam).

→ **Roast uncovered** until brown and tender (about an hour, turning once after 30 minutes).

When you cook non-root veggies such as squash, onions, peppers, or any other vegetable that you choose, make sure that they are cut the same size. They will need less time to cook. If you mix them with the root vegetables, make sure to give the latter a head start; otherwise, you will have some of the non-root veggies overcooked, while the root veggies are undercooked. Remember to use just a quick Pam spray to prevent greasiness. Any left-over veggies can be used in salads, or reheated the next night.

Finding new ways to enjoy the vegetables you need everyday, can really upgrade your healthy food plan. Dense vegetables contain less water, so you can prepare a smaller serving with the same amount of satisfaction. These delicious roasted vegetables can replace some of the old-hat 'white and starchy' foods which can throw off your metabolism.

You will find that adapting these recipes and shopping for the basic food staples you need for healthy eating can be a fun challenge, almost like a game. With proper planning, the same foods that you prepare for dinner can be used the following day for lunch or snacks by following the "Lunch Box" theory.

Additional "Tips" for the Healthy Cook

The most important resource that you could include as an information guidebook is ***The Food Shopping Counter*** **by Annette Natow and Jo-Ann Heslin.** It analyzes the nutrient content of foods. It might be difficult for you to figure out the amount of fiber or sodium in a fresh food like a cantaloupe or cabbage. It features calories, sodium, fiber, fat, carbohydrates, protein, and portion size for all the foods you can buy in a supermarket, including fresh vegetables as well as brand names. Phil McGraw included another similar guide in his ***Ultimate Weight Solution Food Guide.*** **(Pocketbooks)** Such a guide is indispensable to winning your weight war.

Another very helpful resource is the ***Dictionary of Healthful Food Terms*** by Bev Bennett and Virginia Van Vynckt. It provides readable descriptions of any nutritional term you have ever wondered about. This Dictionary appendix even provides some of the benefits of each kind of foods, as well as defining the concerns that health professionals have about additives.

Yogurt ideas: Plain yogurt is very high in protein and low in fat. It can be used to make wonderful cheeses for healthy snacks or to add to other recipes.

Yogurt cheese: Drain 1 quart of low-fat plain yogurt in your large sieve lined with cheesecloth or paper towels. Leave the yogurt to drain for 4 to 8 hours depending on the firmness you want. You can cover it with plastic wrap and keep it in the refrigerator as it drains. Overnight is convenient and works well. For more taste varieties of yogurt cheese, you can season it with salt and herbs of your choosing such as chives, garlic, and pepper. Use it as you would cream cheese to serve with whole grain crackers, to stuff celery, or serve with veggies as a dip (leaving it a little thinner or thin with skim milk to the desired consistency. If you roll it in chives, parsley, herbs or pepper, you can serve it as a cheese ball.

Replace some of the liquid that you drained off with orange or lemon juice, add some natural zest to create the desired thickness, and sweeten with Splenda if you want. You can even add some drops of vanilla and serve with fresh fruit or an All-Fruit spread.

For an absolutely wonderful new product with only *100 calories, 0 grams of fat, 4 grams of fiber and 3 grams of protein,* you must try **Vita Muffins.** They come in a blueberry flavor as well as *chocolate* (absolutely fabulous treat), and can be found in the organic freezer section. **Uncle Sam's Breakfast Bars** are the healthiest, quick, get-up-and-go breakfast bars around. They are made with lots of whole grains, fruits, and minimal amounts of fat and sugar. **Hellman's Canola Mayonnaise** has ½ of the fat (it's the good fat) and it tastes like regular mayonnaise. **Newman's Salad Dressings** are very tasty, can have low to lite fat, and a little goes a long way. **"Dijonnaise"** has 0 grams of fat, and is creamier than mustard alone. It can be found in the condiments section near the mustard. **Non-fat Half and Half** is made by several companies and is very tasty and creamy. Watch the amount you use as it contains some sugar. Remember to buy **non-fat Carnation canned milk** to use in sauces and soups. You really can't taste the difference.

Flat-out wraps can be found in the deli section of the market with lots of fiber, very low carbohydrates, and high protein. Your choices depend on your taste as long as you check the nutrition labels. Use them for pizza crust using your "skinny" marinara sauce and sensible toppings. It's delicious!

Salad Dressings: Marinades

These dressings can be used as both salad dressings and marinades for meats, fish, and poultry.

After the earlier discussions about using dressings to marinate veggies, here is a recipe for homemade dressing and the many varieties I have found very useful for veggies, salads, and as a meat marinade. Very important! Do not use any marinade used on raw meat as a sauce unless you simmer it for at least five minutes when making the sauce. *Marinate fish for no longer than thirty minutes, or the released acid will actually cook the fish!*

Jane's Basic Lite Dressing

→ 1/3 cup **olive oil**

→ 1/3 cup balsamic **vinegar**

→ ½ cup **water**

→ 1 package **Good Seasons Italian Salad Dressing Mix**

→ 1 tablespoon **mustard**

→ Mix well in covered jar and keep in the refrigerator if you don't use it every day. It is best and will keep nicely for a few days at room temperature.

Added flavorings:

→ 1 teaspoon **oregano** and 1 packet of **Splenda** (this takes on a Greek flavoring) or:

→ 1 teaspoon of **curry** powder or:

→ 1 teaspoon of **tarragon** and add white or red **wine vinegar**.

→ 1 tablespoon of **pesto** mixed well with a whisk.

As you can see, the varieties are truly endless, with lots of possibilities with which to experiment. Citrus dressing would be great with fish or salad with fruit in it. Just replace the vinegar with lemon or lime juice and eliminate the mustard.

Fiber Surprises

It is important to examine which foods give us the necessary fiber that we need in our diet. (Twenty-five grams are usually suggested.) It was surprising to discover that salads and veggies are what most people believe will fill the fiber requirements. Fiber not only helps to fill us up, but also has wonderful health benefits for digestion and nutrition. The benefits of fiber have been covered by a multitude of nutrition books. Supplements can help, but make sure that you read the labels and select foods that have the most fiber in them. The following is a list of the foods that was surprising.

- 1 orange – 7 grams

- Whole grain bread – 3 grams

- Old-fashioned oatmeal – 5 grams

- ½ cup red beans – 9 grams

- 1 cup blackberries – 5 grams

- ½ cup cooked spinach – 2 grams

- ½ cup of most fruit – 2 grams

- 1 cup split pea soup – 10 grams

- 1 heaping teaspoon soluble fiber – 5 grams

- ½ cup string beans – 5 grams

Water, Water Everywhere

Water will quench your thirst, flush out your system, and will help your stomach feel comfortable. For some of us, it's hard to drink the recommended eight glasses of water a day. Everywhere you look these days, you can see people carrying around bottles of water. One trick of the trade is to buy twenty-four-ounce bottles of water, and leave one at different settings where you hang out.   If you finish three of them a day, you've done it. Leave one in your car, by the TV, in your work areas, and in the kitchen. If it's there, you will be reminded to drink it.

Planning Appropriately

IF YOU FAIL TO PLAN, YOU WILL PLAN TO FAIL! A very wise person created this logical saying. Planning is essential to your ultimate victory in winning your war on weight. These suggestions are just the beginning. Take the time to explore your creativity and to enjoy your search for all the healthy possibilities in your food preparation. You are the only one who can ensure your success in giving your body the chance to shift into the person you plan to be. This is not a diet! It is a healthy, permanent, lifestyle change.

If you had a child who needed special attention to thrive and survive, you would spend everything you could in order to get the necessary help for him or her. You deserve the same attention and consideration. You are worth it. Your future-self will be delighted. You can enjoy the challenge in a fun-filled way – for the health of your life.

Summary:

While you are altering your beliefs and attitudes about eating and food, changing techniques of food preparation and creating new ways to enjoy your favorite recipes are important. You can stay in control by eating smaller meals more often throughout the day.

Replace refined white flours and sugars with whole grains, high fiber, and lots of vegetables.

Drink at lots of water. Change negative thoughts, attitudes and beliefs into positive affirmations and repeat them often.

Prepare, cook, and enjoy **real** food that is healthy and delicious avoiding the sugars that are included in most mass-produced commercial foods.

Treat yourself to the care you deserve by creating a "lunch box" of healthy, well-balanced food that you can "snack on" all day, with only the desired number of calories for the day. You have the freedom to adapt *your* favorite recipes to your healthy lifestyle. A wonderful source of information is a food guide such as *"The Food Shopping Counter"* or Dr. Phil's *"Ultimate Weight Solution Food Guide"*.

CHAPTER 12

Conclusion: The ABCs of Winning Your Personal Weight War

Winning your weight war requires strategic consideration to getting the outcome you want. Decisions are made about what kinds of food you put into your mouth, how often you eat, and how slowly or quickly you consume the food. You make a serious commitment to how often, how long, and the intensity with which you exercise. In essence you are making a conscious life-style choice. There is room and time for interesting side trips "to smell the roses," so to speak. That allows you to enjoy all the wonderful social opportunities that fill your life with special meaning. As long as you keep your "end" in mind, and get back onto the straight and narrow road of a purposeful and disciplined eating and exercise program, you will achieve your victory. There is no quick or easy way - you are in it for the long haul. The reality is that you have to implement those choices, and keep on putting them into practice for the rest of your life.

As Maria Von Trapp said in **The Sound of Music,** learning to sing is easier when you "start at the very beginning" with the "ABCs." Let's make this conclusion easy to remember by using your own version of the "Weight War ABC's".

A Accept that you already have a multitude of internal resources and experiences of success that you can identify and rely on to take care of yourself with love and care. Make sure you apply these resources to the whole issue of creating a healthy lifestyle with exercise, small quantities, and nutritional food choices.

Belief systems that are empowering and positive will overcome emotional sabotages and temptations. You are entitled to have faith in your personal strengths, commitment, abilities, and confidence to accomplish the goals that you set. You have had many positive experiences which give you the self-assurance to meet any challenges that life throws at you. Believing in yourself is an important positive attitude that can help you to overcome anxieties and frustrations, which generate emotional obstacles.

Create an internal future self as an ally and a reference point to evaluate the importance of your temptations in comparison to your ultimate goals which will help you make appropriate, healthy choices in your own best self-interest.

Determine any 'secondary gains' or positive benefits of staying at your present weight that focuses on what you would miss when you reached your goal weight. These "benefits" would be a roadblock to achieving your smaller size and shape. When you acknowledge and appreciate those benefits that accompany your present weight, it is possible to find even more effective means of satisfying those intentions, so that they will continue to serve the positive functions. Examples of secondary gains that would defeat your best intentions may take the form of mourning the loss of favorite high-calorie foods, equating being a small size with being vulnerable or impotent, or using extra weight as a convenient protection against sexual attentions from others.

Evaluate the benefits of getting to your goal weight. What's in it for you to achieve your goal and maintain it? This is what makes your efforts worthwhile and puts all those fattening foods into a "healthy" perspective and diminishes their importance. Keep those benefits in your conscious awareness by writing them down and posting them anyplace where you make eating decisions. You can carry this list with you when you go to a restaurant or to the grocery store. It may even be helpful to highlight one at a time to pay more attention to it.

F Focus on 'Fist-fullfillment' to know when to stop eating. As long as you remember that your stomach is about the size of your fist, you will have an objective way to determine when you have eaten enough food. Eating nutritious foods that are low in fat will prevent you from adding to your weight.

G Get rid of the "losing" mentality. Losing is a negative and passive word that means being deprived of something. We spend our lives working hard to avoid losses. We enjoy wins and gains as evidence of success. Exploit this to your benefit. Focus intensely on what you have to win or to gain by getting to your goal weight and maintaining it. That makes all the effort that you will be using to insure your success worthwhile. Get hold of the "Guts" or "intestinal fortitude" to have the determination to fulfill your commitment to your future self.

H The "Head" and the "Heart" helps you achieve success. The head tells you the factual information you need, while the heart focuses on your values which help motivate you. Do you connect more with what you want to achieve, or with doing whatever is necessary to avoid a negative outcome that you don't want? Do you evaluate your successes based on objective data, or on your own subjective internal evaluation? Do you focus on a present gratification, or on future benefits or accomplishments that empower you to be at your best? Do you need to follow a strict routine of procedures to succeed, or do you connect more with choices and options? Do you focus on how things generally stay the same, notice even small differences, or do you have an awareness of consistent progress toward your objectives? Knowing your unique style of achieving success will allow you to formulate your outcomes in language that will have the most meaning to you and will be the most effective in winning your struggle to get to your weight or size goals.

I Internalize your "Cheerleader/Coach". Be kind to yourself! The last thing you need is to be badgered or beaten up, especially by you. An internal cheerleader, who can be supportive when you're feeling down, or be enthusiastic when you are doing well, is a wonderful resource to keep you motivated. Remember that a cheerleader encourages the team even, or especially when that team is behind. A coach provides good information, the discipline for working hard to achieve your goal, and a mindset that you have the ability to accomplish anything you want to do.

J Journaling about the foods you eat, and the exercises you do, will give you a tangible record of what you have achieved so far. You can remind yourself of how far you have come when you feel down or unmotivated. Sometimes it is difficult to adequately and comfortably share your successes with others, and having a permanent record on paper or on your computer is an excellent way of demonstrating your progress to yourself and to others. Giving yourself the responsibility to keep this record will allow you to celebrate a victory each day. If you count calories, keeping a record of fats, carbohydrates and protein intakes as you go will allow you to see clearly what you eat to make progress and highlight which foods cause setbacks. If you need a quick review, or if you re-encounter a struggle that you have already solved, keeping relevant newspaper and magazine articles, or even suggestions from friends, will keep you focused on your objectives.

KKeep a commitment to exercise regularly. In addition to generating a highly efficient metabolism which burns off calories quickly and easily, physical exercise strengthens your bones and tones muscles to prevent injury, reduces depression, builds your self esteem, and helps clothes fit better. You can exercise every day by joining a gym, walking, dancing, climbing stairs, playing sports, lifting weights, doing sit-ups, twisting the night away, or bending down to pick up toys, just to name a few options.

LLove yourself - inside your own body. You will believe that you deserve to achieve your goal weight when you truly accept and love the person inside. It is important to emotionally comfort and nurture the insecure, frightened 'inner child' who has few resources to cope with frustrations, criticism, or disappointments in any other way than eating. That small person needs to be encouraged and cheered on rather than criticized or blamed.

MMake sure to set milestones, and celebrate achieving them. Recognize and appreciate those in your life who provide encouragement or who serve as role models. If you partner with others, note their success stories, so you can inspire yourself to continue your journey to fitness.

NNever accept high calorie treats when they are offered just to be polite, or because you think it is expected. Give yourself respect, and others will as well. Express appreciation to the person offering the treat for the kind gesture, or for the trouble that they must have gone to in preparing (or buying) the food, but explain that the weight program that you have committed to would be in jeopardy. If they are inconsiderate enough to pull out the 'guilt card', respond in kind with a statement such as: "I know I can count on you to help me in reaching my weight goal."

Organize and plan your grocery shopping to include healthy foods for every meal, including items for your "lunch box". This is especially helpful when there is only a limited choice of food at work. Most importantly, you can demonstrate to yourself that you are responsible to take care of all your health needs. Organize your kitchen to eliminate foods that will keep you from accomplishing your weight goals.

Past evidence of success in overcoming difficult challenges and getting to positive outcomes in any context can be used to create a similar strategy to continue the success in this most personal war.

Quicken your pace and intensity for doing customary chores to increase and expand your exercise routine everyday. This will allow your fat-burning metabolism to continue to work efficiently. Quiet negative voices or thoughts which tell you why you can't do what you want. Replace "discouraging words' with empowering beliefs.

Remind yourself often of all the benefits you will enjoy when you reach your goal weight. This keeps you motivated and enthusiastic as you look forward to the more important rewards of getting to your goal and maintaining it.

Self-Hypnosis reprograms your old, unconscious eating and exercise habits to incorporate your new commitment to winning your personal weight war. Self-hypnosis is a way of connecting with your higher consciousness and inner resources to reflect your core values, and reinforce your commitment to specific healthy decisions about what to eat, how much of that food to eat, and how often to exercise. Self-acceptance, reassurance and nurturing of that scared 'inner child', renewed determination, positive self-talk, and commitment are the antidotes to failure.

TTake the time to eat s-l-o-w-l-y, which energizes and excites your taste buds to give you all the physical and emotional satisfaction you deserve. When you eat fast, your gustatory, or taste, receptors do not have time to internally sort out and transmit the satisfaction of the different flavor and aroma experiences to your brain. You deprive yourself of all the enjoyment and fulfillment that food is meant to provide.

UUnderstand the need to create a subtle discrimination between sensations of hunger, and those of comfort, which can become signals to know when to eat and even more importantly when to stop. Once you have eaten a fistful of food, you will feel comfortable. You are nourishing your body rather than stretching out your stomach.

VVitamins and minerals are essential to maintaining good health and fitness. Make sure you at least take a good multivitamin every day, in case your choices or quantities of food are lacking, or do not offer enough of the vitamins and minerals you need. Remember that menopausal women particularly need extra calcium to protect their bone strength and prevent osteoporosis.

WWrite down specifically the outcomes that you want to achieve rather than verbalizing the typical kind of general, abstract "New Year's Resolution" such as "I want to lose weight!" It is important to determine the basic values of achieving the weight goal, and how that goal is impacted by the benefits. Record how getting to that weight and maintaining it will be helpful to you. Keep a record of low fat and low calorie recipes that you have found to be effective and delicious or experiment with adapting family recipes to reflect your new commitment to yourself.

XEXtreme fad diets might work in the short term, but it is essential to make permanent lifestyle shifts that honor your highest values to empower effective, long-lasting satisfying changes. EXercise with the same enthusiasm that you used to invest in eating.

YYou are the only one who has total control over choosing the quality and the quantity of foods that you put into your mouth, as well as how much you exercise. You are the only one who is responsible for making sure your "future self" is brought to reality.

ZZero in on the emotional needs that drive your eating behavior. You often confuse hunger for food with hungers to relieve emotional stress such as loneliness, boredom, frustration, anger or disappointment. It is important and possible to discover alternatives to satisfying these hungers in more effective ways than eating food.

When you talk about the exit strategy in this weight war you must remember that like any victor, you must maintain control of the conquered territory – *your new waistline and body*. Since you know how to achieve success, you have strategies that help maintain it. If you slide back, or indulge a little too heavily, you can be more restrictive until you get yourself back on track. It's not about 'never'. You will enjoy high calorie foods from time to time. The trick is to plan for that so it becomes a purposeful treat, rather than one of desperation or habit. Your ultimate success is like a thermostat, in that it will fluctuate back and forth around the weight you have set for yourself. Your strength is that **you** are in control of regulating that thermostat. That is the true measure of someone who is a winner in this weight war. Keep reinforcing your commitment to stay in control of your weight. Exercise regularly – and often and your body will continue to take care of you for a very long time.

Take the opportunity to celebrate even the small victories in your daily battles, so you can become proud of all your efforts as you watch your continued progress toward achieving and maintaining all the benefits that you want for yourself in winning the war on your weight.

Appendices

I. Create a Future Self

↪ Imagine a visual image of your "future self."

↪ What does it look like?

↪ Where do you see it in your mind's eye?

↪ Does it appear to be very close to you or far away?

↪ Can you see your whole body—including the expression on your face?

↪ What are you wearing that gives you pleasure?

↪ Is this image in color or black and white?

↪ Is it fuzzy or in focus?

↪ Can you see a background in that picture?

↪ Is the image panoramic or framed?

↪ Discover if it is a moving picture or a still.

↪ How far in the future is that image?

↪ Is there a sound track or is it silent?

↪ How do you feel when you look at that picture?

"Make this visual representation of your future self real, bright, vivid, colorful, focused, three dimensional, panoramic, and three to five feet away. Make sure there is a sound track in your image. Tell that future self all that it means to you to bring her into reality and for you to in-habit that body. Make a commitment to that future self at your high-est value that you will do whatever you need to do to bring that future self into reality. More than any other person in the universe, he or she is completely dependent on your food decisions for his or her very ex-istence, from this moment into forever. You have a natural ally in this metaphorical image. When you use this as a criterion for making those decisions, you reinforce your commitment and increase the likelihood that you will be successful. The concept of having another cheerleader on your side is very empowering. You never seem to have enough posi-tive cheers to be 'encouraging' (giving you *courage* to go down the path you have chosen). The test is to make a determination of which is worth more to you: eating that cookie or getting to your future self."

11. Goal Weight Questionnaire

1. As a child or an adolescent, were you ever teased about your weight?

2. Were many family members overweight?

3. What was the conventional wisdom in your family about food and eating as you grew up? For example, was there an inherent value in being a member of the "clean plate club"?

4. Were you made to stay at the table until <u>all</u> your "vegetables were eaten"?

5. Was having enough to eat an ongoing problem, or was abundant food spoiling or going to waste?

6. Has your social life ever been affected by your weight?

7. Are you presently involved in an occupation that requires or encourages you to maintain a certain weight?

8. What does being at your goal weight, and maintaining it at that level do for you that makes having it important and worthwhile?

9. How will you behave differently when you have reached your goal weight than you do now?

10. In your mind's eye, make an image of yourself as you are right now, as if you were looking at yourself in a mirror, or as someone else would see you. How do you feel inside when you see that image?

11. Have there been any benefits or "gains" that have accompanied your present weight? (What would you miss by being at your goal weight?)

12. Can you identify anything in your personal experience that would prevent you from accomplishing your goal?

13. In your mind, what is something in your life that you wanted to do very much, and achieved, even if it took you a long time?

14. What was the evidence to you that you were successful?

15. Did you ever become discouraged in getting that outcome?

16. As you think about all that effort, would you be willing to do it all over again from the beginning?

17. Is there anything about going to all that effort that would make maintaining it easier than having to do it all again?

18. Are there any foods that you absolutely wouldn't eat?

19. What are foods that your future self would never put in her body?

III. Mental Rehearsal for Self-Esteem

Think back to any past situation in which your success is undeniable. Ask yourself the following six questions:

1. What were the first steps that allowed you to initiate that process?

2. What *images* came to mind at that moment of time?

3. What did you *say* to yourself to make that outcome happen?

4. What *sensations* or feelings did you experience, which let you know this outcome was worth the effort it would take to achieve it?

5. What encouragement did you need when the necessary work became challenging, bogged down, or boring?

6. How did you know that you had finally arrived at that success?

What behaviors were essential to that success?

1. Notice the qualities of the image itself. (Are you seeing yourself as if it were a video or are you seeing everything through your own eyes? Is it large or small? Bright or dim? Moving or still? Color or black and white? Close or distant? Flat or three dimensional? Framed or panoramic?)

2. Notice the sounds and what you say to yourself in your memory of that scene. (Voices, sounds, direction of sounds, volume of sounds, rhythm/flat, speed, tonality of voice, quality of sound)

3. Imagine you can step inside that scene, and feel what that success feels like in your body. (Notice whether they are warm or cool, smooth or rough-edged, light or heavy.)

4. Mentally rehearse a scene of your next challenge in the same way you just thought about your success. Make sure the scene of that challenge matches up those same visual and sound qualities as your successful memory. (Create and edit the video as you go along.) Watch yourself easily and confidently getting your goal.

5. When you are satisfied with the inner film you have created, step inside it in your imagination. Feel those feelings. Compare this movie – and feeling with those of that positive memory you recalled. Is it at least as vivid and satisfying? Does it look truly inviting and gratifying?

6. Notice any differences from the memory that detract from it being satisfying or appropriate. If any aspect needs to be modified, step out of the scene and make any adjustments. Add elements or adjust the sound or the picture until it looks and feels intensely desirable. Step back in and check it again.

7. You can now re-energize your good feelings with an new determination, knowing you have done it successfully before.

(Adapted from "New Behavior Generator" with permission from Midlantic Institute of NLP.)

IV. Evaluating Your Hunger

Take stock of, chew over, or size up what is really generating the sensations you interpret as hunger.

→ Thirst often masquerades as hunger. Drinking water, seltzer, tea, or even coffee may be as filling and satisfying as any food.

→ You may be "hungry" for interesting activity or a challenge to relieve boredom.

→ Perhaps you are "hungering" for the company of friends. It is sad to say that mere food is not the solution. If you eat, you are still in need of companionship to feel satisfied.

→ Another emotion that often masquerades as physical hunger is sadness. It's when you revert to your first source of comfort and connection with others—eating.

→ Stress from demands made by others, or even demands for perfection from inside of us, generates an uncomfortable tension. Eating just delays the pressure to perform.

→ •When you eat brainlessly, without thinking, you are eating because you become enslaved to a habit of eating at a certain time or in certain situations. It is generally unrelated to whether or not you are actually hungry.

→ •Sometimes you eat because you don't want to be told what to do—even if you, yourselves, are the ones doing the telling.

→ •Family expectations: "Clean Plate Club" or "You can't have dessert until you eat all your vegetables." This drives the habit of eating past your comfort level.

↪ •Snacking or tasting while cooking can really pack on the calories since you then go and eat a "normal" meal when it is ready, even though your stomach might be signaling that you have had enough.

↪ •Stomach growling is the natural contraction that your stomach makes on its way to recapturing those fist-sized dimensions. I like to think of it as nature's method of non-invasive bariatric surgery.

↪ •Learn to recognize your natural signs of physical hunger. It is not accidental that the first meal of the day is known as "break fast" because it breaks your overnight fast. Assuming you have not eaten in twelve hours, you can experience a normal hunger in the morning.

↪ •Eating very slowly allows us to monitor and evaluate how close to comfortable you can get while at the same time enjoying the taste of everything you eat.

V. Hunger Chart

When to start eating – When to stop

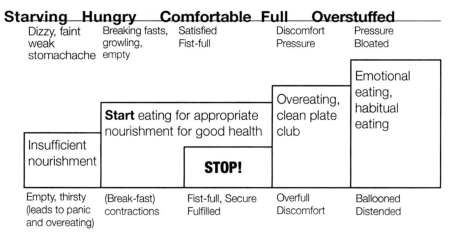

Starving	Hungry	Comfortable	Full	Overstuffed
Dizzy, faint weak stomachache	Breaking fasts, growling, empty	Satisfied Fist-full	Discomfort Pressure	Pressure Bloated

| | | | Overeating, clean plate club | Emotional eating, habitual eating |

Start eating for appropriate nourishment for good health

Insufficient nourishment

STOP!

| Empty, thirsty (leads to panic and overeating) | (Break-fast) contractions | Fist-full, Secure Fulfilled | Overfull Discomfort | Ballooned Distended |

VI. Overcoming the Temptation Battle

1. Think of a specific time when you felt upset about some emotional issue that compelled you to eat or tempted you to eat something you didn't want.

2. Run a thirty second "movie" in your mind's eye to represent that incident. It could be the most recent time or perhaps the most intense circumstance when you were ready to give up on your goals.

3. Arbitrarily rank that negative feeling that occurs in response to that movie as a ten on a scale of one to ten.

4. With each step in this exercise, you will be asked to change some aspect of how this "movie" is presented in your mind's eye. The fun is to discover how the negativity is reduced, and how your enthusiasm and motivation for honoring your commitment to "win" this war is enhanced in response to these changes.

5. Run the movie *twice as fast* in only fifteen seconds. Stop! Notice how much lower the negative feelings seem.

6. Run the movie *backwards*. Stop! How low does ranking become now?

7. Think of your favorite comedy show such as the *I Love Lucy* or *Seinfeld* series. Now bring to mind the funniest episode you can think of: such as the time Lucy and Ethel were in the candy factory stuffing the pieces of candy in their pockets, aprons, mouths; anyplace they could find rather than letting them fall on the floor. Or the image of George Castanza eating a piece of cake from the garbage can in the kitchen, or worrying about a way to regrow his hair. This time, run your original movie to the middle, *insert the funny scene,* and

then finish your movie. Stop, and take stock of how much the negativity has been reduced.

8. Run the movie *adding circus music* until the end. Stop! Rank the negative feelings now.

9. *Now* run the original thirty-second movie again, and discover how all those feelings have shifted once again. It should be close to one, or even zero.

10. Refocus your awareness in vivid color on your *future self,* who represents all the advantages of getting to and maintaining your goal weight, and remind yourself of how much value and significance you assign to this outcome. *(Adapted from the "Pattern Interruption" intervention with permission from Midlantic Institute of NLP, Silver Spring, Maryland.)*

VII. Self-Hypnosis Introduction

- Self-hypnosis is a relaxed, highly suggestible state wherein suggestions can be directed to the self. Since it is a learned, conditioned response, it needs to be practiced as much as possible for the best outcome.

- You can reorient to the present alert state with specific suggestions for a time limit to the experience or a prearranged cue with suggestions for feeling alert, refreshed and relaxed when your eyes open.

- You can be assured that should an emergency occur, you will be instantly responsive and alert.

- Spontaneous development of complete amnesia during self-hypnosis is impossible. Partial amnesia may occur relative to your own personal style or habit of forgetting or remembering.

- Specific suggestions may take the form of choosing healthy foods such as: vegetables, lean meats, low fat and low sugar foods; exercising regularly; eating slowly; finding satisfaction with a fistful of food; or recognizing emotional conflicts as distinct from hunger.

- For your protection, you can suggest to yourself that no one can hypnotize you by any means, without your specific permission and cooperation.

- Be sure to end each practice session with the suggestion that you will go into hypnosis more easily and quickly each time you desire to do so.

- You may suggest that self-hypnosis can merge with actual

sleep if done at bedtime. You will awake in the morning feeling refreshed and alert.

→ Make sure you reorient yourself with suggestions to be alert, energized and refreshed. Shake your hands, tap your feet on the floor, stretch your arms, move your head on your shoulders, take a deep breath and say aloud in a firm voice: *Alert, Refreshed, and Energized.*

→ You may make an audio-tape with all the instructions to experience hypnosis and include the specific suggestions that you have created for yourself, while you feel relaxed and comfortable. In that way you can create one set of suggestions to use at night, and another set to use during the day. You have the flexibility to change it as you make progress.

VIII. Eight Steps to Self-Hypnosis

1. Plan your suggestions first. Keep them stated in the positive. Connect these positive suggestions with visual symbols or representations.

2. Recall specific times when you felt calm, relaxed secure and competent. Imagine you are actually there. Think of a specific word that will bring this to mind.

3. Take a deep breath in and hold it. Look up as far as you can as if you were looking up at your forehead. Now with your eyes looking up, close your eyelids. Now allow your eyes to relax down toward your cheekbone as you slowly breathe out.

Or:

Allow your eyes to focus on a high spot in the room. You will be counting down, silently from five to one as you relax progressively. As your eyes begin to defocus, take a deep breath and let it out slowly and think "five." As your eyes begin to get heavy and close, think "four." As you can feel your muscles in your chest, shoulders and arms relax think "three." As you can feel the muscles in your stomach and abdomen relax think "two." As you take another deep breath and let it out *very* slowly, and continue to experience increased comfort, think "one"—and thoroughly enjoy this gift that you give yourself.

4. Deepen the experience with the recalled relaxation imagery. As you continue to breathe easily and deeply, you can tell yourself that you will feel more and more relaxed with each breath that you take.

5. Now imagine that you are in the context that you want to see yourself. Insert the positive suggestions and imagery that you

constructed before you started, and see yourself, in vivid color and clear focus, behaving differently in the future.

6. Return to relaxation and comfort imagery.

7. Make post-hypnotic suggestions as to specifically how you want to feel when you open your eyes. If you counted down to one, make sure you count back up to five to reorient. If you are taking a break in the middle of the day, you will suggest to yourself that you will feel refreshed, relaxed and alert when you open your eyes. If you are using it to help you sleep at night, you can suggest that this relaxation will take you into a natural, deep and restful sleep, and that you will wake in the morning refreshed and alert.

8. Reorient completely by patting your hands on your lap, tapping your feet, stretching your arms and shoulders, taking a deep breath, and saying out loud: ***"Refreshed, Energized, and Alert".***

(Adapted from the "Self- Hypnosis" pattern with permission from the Midlantic Institute of NLP, Silver Spring, Maryland.)

IX. A Complete Hypnosis Script

Hypnosis is a way for you to become familiar with yourself at another level of being, and you've known **all along** that you can learn while you're relaxed. I just wonder whether your conscious mind is aware of what you are wanting to discover about going into a delightful trance, ... and what your unconscious mind already knows about the wonderful potentials, ... and has already relaxed into a productive trance of learnings and understandings necessary to growth, ... and I don't know whether your unconscious would choose a light trance, or a **deep trance** or a *medium trance* to do that important work, but I do know that everyone finds their own speed to go into a trance as well as the right degree of trance for them. So, you can use my words, suggestions and ideas as a stimulus for you to do you're own thinking.

You probably already noticed that your face muscles are relaxed and that your breathing is slower than it was. That's because you are doing it exactly the right way, and since you and your brain are the boss of your body, you can even make your relaxation even more than it already is, because our bodies already know how to relax. We relax a little bit more each time we breathe out. So to help relax even more, just take a slow, deep relaxing breath all the way in and as you slowly breathe out through your mouth, say R-E-L-A-X to yourself in your inside thinking and feel your body let loose of tension.

The brain is the master control of the body. You can think anything you want and your emotions and physical sensations respond to what you think and believe inside. You can be a "Winner from the Inside Out!"

Your unconscious may begin to notice a calm quiet place, a peace, a sense of comfort, relaxation, and safety, as you learn more and more about your ability to relax thoroughly and completely as this special place in your unconscious awareness becomes more and more vivid, surrounded with an effortless calm, comfortable peace, and a place of complete relaxation and security.

Be there! Seeing what you see, hearing what you hear, and feeling the sensations and emotions, which are **there** in that safe, secure, relaxed place that you have created in your imagination.

Your unconscious mind can allow my words to form meanings, images, sensations, and thoughts, which come to mind; and are relevant and appropriate to your needs, wants, and desires.

That unconscious mind contains a vast universe of learnings and meaningful experiences with an infinite amount of wisdom. All these important learnings have slipped into your unconscious mind, where they can be used and enjoyed automatically.

And while I have been speaking, your unconscious may have noticed that your respiration has slowed, your blood pressure has lowered, and your muscle tone has changed. You can feel the comfort, inside, as you continue to relax more and more with every breath that you take.

And now imagine the actual sensations of personal accomplishment you will experience when you have reached your goal. It is your unconscious mind that forms that feeling, creates the image and helps you generate that positive energy of you being the best you can be.

You've been **waiting** a long time to make a change in the structure of your body. There is a part of you who will exercise your right to have the body you want, along with sizeable quantities of confidence, hefty portions of esteem, and large helpings of determination. **The difference between success and failure in getting and maintaining control over weight is a 'winning' mindset rather than a 'losing' mentality.**

You can, and will commit yourself to be more fit, more attractive, more energetic, more vivacious you – the real you!

In the past, you may have come to think of yourself as heavy, overweight, or unattractive. It is important that you now change the way that you think of yourself - this is as important as changing your eating habits. Picture yourself being at your goal weight, weighing what you want, as if you had just come out of the shower standing in front of a full length mirror. See your reflection in the mirror – fit, slender, and attractive.

"That is your future self. To bring her into your reality, she is completely dependent <u>for her very existence</u> on all the decisions that you make about what kinds of food you will put in your mouth as well as determining how much of that food to eat from this moment on to forever. Think about how often physical exercise will be part of your life. Make that image as vivid and real as you can, and if it is important enough for you to want it in your future, it will <u>pull</u> you into it.

You want an image which is **appropriate to your age**, *and created as a goal <u>yet to be achieved</u>. In your imagination, make sure you see that image from head to toe, paying special attention to the facial expressions. Now, one at a time, make sure that image is:*

- → life-sized

- → three dimensional

- → clearly focused

- → in vivid color

- → a movie rather than a still picture

- → Panoramic

➥ Free of a particular situation or context, so it is available to you at any time

Now, I invite you to mentally step inside that future self, …. Feel all the sensations that you experience inside that <u>new</u> you. … Imagine what you will feel, think and see as you move around inside that body, weighing what she weighs, and looking at the world through her eyes. Pay particular attention to how she evaluates her food choices and how much she wants to eat."

Now experience how very light you feel without all that unnecessary weight. Tell yourself that you can, and will, look and feel like this because **this** is the real you, which has been hidden and imprisoned by excess weight,   and reconnect with your present self.

"Spend a moment of time inside, now, just enjoying the possibility of that future. …….

Now, I invite you to make a <u>commitment</u> to that future self in your own words, from the very "bottom of your heart" to do whatever it takes to bring her into reality. It is between you and what you imagine that you will look like when you reach your goal weight. This commitment must be taken very seriously by you, because it is made at the level of your highest values, based on what is <u>genuinely</u> important to you. It becomes almost a "covenant" for you with that future self. Notice the response. ……… Take as long as you need, to know that commitment is made."

"Ask that future self to be your ally in helping you make all the wise decisions about the food you eat. The fact is, <u>she</u> has already succeeded in accomplishing that goal. She can remind you of all of those important benefits that you identified that were important about getting to that weight, and maintaining it. Make sure she is willing to take on that role.

"You can allow her to be a guide and your coach to help you make choices about what you put into your mouth to eat. Put an image of your favorite dessert (say its cheesecake) in one hand, and that image of your future self, in the other. Which seems more appetizing to you? Which one would you go for?"

"Now think of another of those temptations that would sabotage your commitment, and compare eating that --- with having the benefits of your future self."

"This is the key to making positive choices. Keep that future self in front of you. Remember that nothing goes into your mouth without making that comparison. Use all the resolve and determination that goes along with that image to be all the encouragement in the world that you need, to make that image real. …….. Now, take a moment of time to determine if you are feeling deprived in any way after making those decisions."

Haven't you waited long enough to gain the pleasure of looking the way you want? – the pleasure of knowing you are taking care of your body, the pleasure of saying 'No Thank You' to temptations which would derail your dreams? Having the pleasure of exercising your right to have the body you deserve? You don't have to wait any longer!"

There are so many rewards and benefits that you have promised yourself when you reach your victory over the excess weight. It is time to be firm, resolute and persistent to honor your future self and prevent "falling into temptation". Chase away the "enemy agents" that would pull you over to the "dark side." See clearly all the beautiful clothes that you will be wearing. Feel the pride, confidence, and esteem that your self-concept will enjoy much more thoroughly than a brief taste in your mouth that quickly goes away.

Before you begin eating, wait a few moments to observe your food. Notice for colors and textures. Inhale deeply, and enjoy any aromas. When you are ready to begin eating, take only small bites of food, and place only small portions on your fork, your spoon, or that food that you hold in your hand such as a sandwich. You will develop the ability to become an ultimate gourmet who is discriminating about what kind of food, and how much of it, you choose to put in your mouth.

Focus your complete attention on the food you are eating. SLOW DOWN! Notice how all the taste buds on your tongue are stimulated by each tiny bit of food. Pay attention to all the flavors, tastes, and textures of the food.

Chew your food thoroughly, and move that good food around in your mouth slowly with your tongue as if it were in slow motion before finally swallowing. By doing this you will satisfy all the taste buds on your tongue, and obtain greater pleasure from your food enjoying each mouthful to its maximum extent. Each time that you swallow, focus your attention on any feelings and sensations in your stomach as you evaluate how close to comfortable you can feel.

As you continue eating you will feel comfortable … completely satisfied … and relaxed until your next meal. Your stomach is just about the size of your fist. Make an image in your mind's eye of your fist. Notice how relatively small, that fist is. As you continue to eat slowly, you can feel that comfort and satisfaction with that fist full of food. Feel that "fist-full-filling" feeling.

Let yourself feel ever increasing feelings of comfort in your stomach so that when you finished eating a "fistfull of food", you have a "fist-full-fill-ing feeling" of comfort and satisfaction with each taste of food. Take in the feeling of comfortable fullness each time that you swallow.

Tell yourself that time is slowing down, and there's lots of time. Each second is stretching it out; far, far out. Notice how, as you eat, there's so much time between each bite that you take and as you chew your food slowly,…. notice how you feel as if every second is a minute, …. and that there's so much time, as if everything is in slow motion.

When you eat slowly enough, you can be recognize the sensations of feeling comfortable, and be satisfied with smaller amounts of food so your stomach will no longer be stretched out.

When, at last, you can enjoy the feelings of comfortable and complete satisfaction in that "fist-full" of food, as if you have been eating for hours, you might be totally surprised to find out how much of that food is left on your plate.

You can make sure that you only eat enough food to be comfortable. You will want to be a tightwad about the fat in your food. If you are not stingy about the fat you eat, those calories and excess food are **"going to waste on your waist." "The essence of that waste is to take *more* of what you want less of."**

Exercise, movement, and exertion, with intensity, burn off calories. You can almost feel the sensation as your body responds to this increased motion … as the muscles produce that metabolic heat which consumes the fat your body had stored. Feeling the release of energy … as it flows inside your body …. Moving you to move, moving you to imagine your body, bones, and muscles, as they become stronger and stronger, … healthier and healthier, … your shape shifting, tightening, firming, and fit; as your body works to dissolve the excess fat and calories, … feeling the increased **warmth, satisfaction**

and pride of taking charge of your body with strength, caring, and responsibility.

Now, I am going to stop talking, and invite you to take all the time in the world that you need in the next 30 seconds of clock time to be with yourself, for yourself, by yourself, inside of yourself to appreciate yourself for all that good work you are doing for yourself – so that the **winds of change can inspire and empower you** to make all the changes you want – now....

Understanding that you have done important work for yourself, feeling comfortable, and satisfied with your decision to nourish and nurture yourself with responsibility and caring, to develop an awareness of thinking differently about the whole issue of **gaining all the benefits you want by being at your goal weight – Feeling the pleasure of eating less is more and more satisfying, ... to focus on having the body you desire; and you don't have to wait any longer to exercise your ability and your right ---- to gain the body you want, that makes all this effort worthwhile.** Notice all the changes you can make – later on, as you begin to use more and more of these ideas, thoughts and commitments to get to the weight you want.

You can exercise your right to feel fulfilled with that fist-full-fillment of food, when you can take pride in your decision to enjoy large amounts of self-confidence, as you enjoy small amounts of food to nourish you completely.

The entire experience can seem like a dream, remembered and forgotten, real and imagined, as your unconscious mind protects your conscious awareness so that what seems like a short time becomes a long time; ... and what seemed a long time is really no time at all. Now, if you wish, you can continue to relax into a deep, satisfying sleep, full of empowering and comforting dreams,…….. and awaken thoroughly rested in the morning.

Or you can choose to think about your everyday conscious world, knowing you can repeat this good exercise as often as you wish.

Wiggle your fingers, tap your toes, move your head slowly around. Rotate your shoulders, stretch your arms out, think about the room you are in.

Say aloud: **Alert, refreshed, and energized**, open you eyes, and get on with your day.

(You may purchase CD's of this hypnosis script available at www. wintheweightwar.com)

X. IDEAS FOR HEALTHY RECIPES
by Jane Mercado

Fish in Packets
4 servings cooked at 400 degrees F.
- **Tilapia** *or your favorite fish*
- *1* **lemon** *sliced thinly*
- *1 teaspoon dried* **dill** *and/or* **tarragon**
- *4* **green onions** *cut in long shreds*
- **Butter spray**
- *Heavy duty foil or parchment paper*

→ Tear off 14 inches of foil or paper for each packet.

→ Spray generously with butter spray.

→ Place fish in the center and season each piece with salt and pepper to taste.

→ Decorate the fish with lemon slices and green onions.

→ Sprinkle herbs on top.

→ Bring sides together to make packets, sealing the four sides.

→ Place on the cookie sheet.

→ Bake in pre-heated oven 15 minutes, check for flakiness or doneness.

→ It's important not to overcook the fish. Remember that it will continue to cook in the packet a bit as well.

→ Serve packets on a serving dish and invite guests to open them carefully.

This technique can be used for poultry as well, and keeps lean cuts tender and juicy if you don't overcook them. You might want to change the herbs, and add garlic to the poultry.

Three Crock Pot recipes

As with the other tools of cooking, I find the crock pot to be the most helpful and healthy. There are many books on the subject and you can adapt the recipes to meet your healthy desires. There are tricks to using the crock pot, so following the manufacturer's directions about fluids and how the crock pot works most efficiently are important. The way you layer the food in the pot is important. Thicken the sauce with a mix of 3 tablespoons flour with ¼ cup cold liquid after you have removed the solids. Turn on high and cook until it thickens. Like many gravies, you can adjust the amount of flour according to how much of the natural juices are left in the pot,

Chili

Using your favorite chili recipe, just cut out the fat by buying very lean meat and using less of it with the other ingredients. For instance, use twice the beans with the same amount of tomatoes. The **chili packs by McCormick's** *with the proportions they recommend work very well. Include chopped* **onions, garlic,** *and* **green peppers.** *(Frozen veggies are OK.) You can increase the seasonings and flavors while you lower the fat content. Beans are wonderful complete carbohydrates and work well with protein, lots of fiber and other nutrients.*

White Chili

Change the meat from beef to chicken breast ground meat and use white beans. This is a little different, and is also delicious. Remember to be creative. If you use curry powder instead of the chili packet, you can "invent" curry chili. Add your own favorite seasoning along with the curry powder. Have fun! Add a can of chunk pineapple (drained of juice) with the curry chili and jalapeno peppers. You will be delighted.

Tenderloin Pork with Fruit

- ↪ Cut a package of tenderloins in half, (usually 2 per package) so you have 4 pieces.

- ↪ Season the pork on both sides with garlic salt and pepper to taste.

- ↪ In your pot, layer the following:

- ↪ 1 package frozen chopped **onions** or 1 whole onion

- ↪ 1 cup mixed **dried fruit**

- ↪ Add meat to the pot on top of the onions and fruit.

- ↪ Add ½ cup water, broth, or white wine.

- ↪ Finally put the contents of one can of celery soup, undiluted on top of the meat.

- ↪ Cover, cook for 6–8 hours, or until very tender. It is important to leave on the cover for the entire cooking time, or the heat will be reduced and it will take longer to cook.

- ↪ Serve with a small amount of brown rice or spaghetti squash.

Spaghetti Squash *is easy to prepare. Heat oven to 350 degrees for 45 minutes ahead of time and place halved pieces on sprayed cookie sheet, cut side down. Cook until tender. You can test for doneness when a kitchen fork can pierce the skin after 30 minutes. Leave on the cookie sheet until you are ready to serve. Carefully turn over each piece, and scrape the fleshy inside with a fork. You will see that it falls onto the plate in spaghetti like shreds. Season with a little butter and/or salt to your taste*

Lamb Kabob with Rosemary:

- *Boneless* **leg of lamb** *or shoulder 1/3 pound per person*
- *2 cups* **Buttermilk** *(or sweet milk with 1 T. vinegar*
- *2 large cloves of* **garlic**, *chopped*
- *2 t. crushed dried* **rosemary**
- *1 red* **onion**

   ↪ Cube **meat** to 1 ½ inch squares

   ↪ Mix next 4 ingredients to make a marinade, cover and refrigerate for 2-4 hours.

   ↪ Cut onion into quarters, separate the slices.

   ↪ Heat the grill according to directions after spraying with Pam.

   ↪ Drain the meat, and alternating with slices of onions, put on skewers.

   ↪ Set the skewers on paper towels and season with garlic salt and pepper to taste.

   ↪ Grill 3-5 minutes per side or until it has reached the desired doneness.

   ↪ Serve on top of your favorite green salad.

Lasagna without Pasta
**(Serves 4 persons in 8 x 8 oven proof dish
baked at 350 degrees for 45 minutes)**

You can use our family's favorite recipe for this dish and others; just substitute grilled vegetables for the pasta. Reduce the quantity of sauce by 1 cup, considering that without pasta to soak up the sauce, it would be too liquid. You can make fabulous chicken spaghetti sauce by leaving out the beef, and using ground chicken breast instead. Ground turkey is great as well. I use low fat cheese and spice it up with lots of garlic, oregano, basil and low-fat ricotta cheese.

→ Put ½ cup thick meat sauce in bottom of pan.

→ Layer grilled vegetables to cover the sauce.

→ (Make ricotta cheese spread by adding garlic salt, pepper and one egg to 3 cups ricotta cheese and 4 tablespoons grated Parmesan cheese).

→ Layer the one half of the cheese spread over the vegetables and sprinkle with low-fat cheese like mozzarella.

→ Repeat the layers and bake in the pre-heated oven for 45 minutes, or until golden and bubbling.

→ Remove from oven and let it cool for 10 minutes before serving. Serve with additional parmesan cheese. (A little cheese goes a long way—so use it judiciously)

→ Serve with a green salad.

Spaghetti Sauce with Spaghetti Squash

- *Use olive oil Pam (or another low fat cooking spray) and sauté one medium onion*
- *Add one pound of ground poultry breast meat and brown.*
- *Add 3 cloves chopped garlic.*
- *Salt and pepper to taste*
- *Add 1 tablespoon each of: oregano, basil.*
- *1 teaspoon Splenda*
- *1 large can of drained, chopped tomatoes.*
- *Simmer over low heat until it thickens, stirring occasionally.*
- *Be creative in adding other flavoring you like in your sauce such as anchovies, olives, peppers, or red wine. (Make sure you cook it down so it isn't too wet.)*
- *Simmer for 20 minutes or to desired consistency.*

- Cut spaghetti squash in half, place on sprayed cookie sheet—cut side down.

- Bake in oven at 350 degrees for 30 minutes or until tender.

- When ready to serve, take a fork and scrape the squash out as it falls into spaghetti-like strings.

- Serve with sauce and Parmesan cheese.

Frittata (Italian Omelet)
Preheat oven to 325 degrees; 8 x 8 inch oven proof pan to serve 4 people

- 2–3 cups leftover cooked vegetables (or your favorites). I prefer to use 1 small, frozen, box of **chopped spinach,** thawed and drained.

- Add **onions and seasonings** of your choice to the veggies and put in the bottom of the dish.

➥ In a separate bowl, mix **egg substitute** to equal 8 eggs, ½ cup **salsa**, and ½ cup **parmesan or feta** cheese. Pour over the vegetables.

➥ **Bake for 30 minutes, or until it is set**

➥ Test by inserting a clean table knife in the middle and see if it comes out clean. If it jiggles, leave in for ten more minutes, and then test again.

➥ Cut into 9 squares. Keep leftovers in the refrigerator covered and reheat in microwave.

➥ Top with more salsa if desired. This keeps for a few days, and is a quick and healthy hot dish, great with salad or marinated veggies.

Broccoli with Sesame Ginger

➥ Steam 1 bag of frozen **broccoli**, and drain

➥ While it cools, toast ¼ cup **sesame seeds** in a small skillet

➥ Toss with **Newman's Sesame Ginger Low-Calorie** dressing just to lightly coat

➥ Serve at room temperature, or cover and refrigerate to serve cold on a hot summer day.

Cucumber and Dill

➥ Thinly slice 1 European **cucumber** and 1 medium **onion**

➥ Layer in bowl, seasoning each layer with **garlic, salt and pepper** to taste

➥ In a separate small bowl, mix ¼ cup **rice vinegar** with 1 package **"Splenda"** and 1 t. **dried dill weed**

➥ Toss, cover and let marinate for at least 2 hours in the refrigerator.

Three-Bean Salad (without sugar or fat)

- *1 can* **each,** *drained:* **Green Beans, Yellow String Beans, Red Kidney Beans**
- *2 packages* **Splenda**
- *Slice 1 medium* **onion**
- *¼ cup* **Rice Vinegar**
- *1 tablespoon* **garlic salt** *and ½ teaspoon* **pepper**

➥ Toss, cover, refrigerate to let it marinate for at least 2 hours before serving.

Black Bean and Corn Salad

(This has always been a family favorite. It takes a little longer to organize the ingredients, but the rave reviews will convince you that it's worth it.)

- *1 can each, rinsed and drained:* **Black Beans, Corn,**
- *1 chopped medium* **onion**
- *1 chopped European* **Cucumber**
- *6 Roma* **Tomatoes** *cubed*
- *½ cup* **Cilantro,** *roughly chopped*
- *1 teaspoon* **garlic salt**
- *½ tablespoon* **pepper**
- *1* **red,** *1* **orange bell pepper** *chopped*
- *Juice of 2 large* **limes**
- *1 tablespoon of either: a) chopped* **pickled jalapeno chili,** *b)* **hot sauce** *to taste, c) fresh* **jalapeno chili** *(available in the "Mexican" section of your supermarket)*

➥ Toss, cover and chill at least 2 hours or more.

Smoothies

- *In the blender, put ½ cup unflavored yogurt*
- **1** *cup crushed ice or small ice cubes (You can also use frozen fruit instead of ice for a very rich taste)*
- *A drop of vanilla or favorite flavoring (a little goes a long way)*
- *A dash of salt*
- *1 cup of your favorite fruit*

  ↪ **Blend and enjoy!** (This recipe makes 2 servings to share or to store in the refrigerator or freezer for later)

Baked Fruit

Apple-banana "pie" *is common in my kitchen because these fruits are always in my fruit basket.*

  ↪ **Spray** a pie plate with low fat cooking spray such as "Pam"

  ↪ **Arrange** the cut-up apple slices in layers (with the healthy skin on) alternating with a layer of sliced bananas

  ↪ **Sprinkle each layer** with a mixture of Splenda and ground cinnamon until filled to the top.

  ↪ **Bake** at 350 for about an hour. It will cook down and become thicker. Check to make sure it stays moist. It will be chewy and smell just like pie. This recipe serves six.

Pineapple-lime combo **is a favorite flavor combination**

  ↪ Using 1 small **sugar-free Lime Jell-O,** follow directions **minus ½ cup water.**

  ↪ **Dissolve**, and put in one small can of **crushed pineapple, drained** (saving the juice for a smoothie)

  ↪ **Stir, cover and chill**

> ↪ **Serve in squares** with a dab of low calorie mayonnaise on top or with low fat whipped topping

The average serving would be 4 x 4 inches. Experiment with other flavors and fruits, and dabs of yogurt to replace the whipped topping. Another possibility is to add the yogurt to the recipe itself, making it creamy.

Fruit Salsa

What a delicious, healthy, savory option to replace rich gravies or sauces!

> ↪ **Chop and peel 4 peaches**

> ↪ Add the juice of **1 lime** and 1 tablespoon of **chopped jalapeno pepper**

> ↪ Mix in a handful of **chopped cilantro** or **parsley** along with 1 chopped **green onion** (or 2 tablespoons **chopped onion**).

Try it on poultry or fish. You can use any fruit with the same combinations of ingredients. If you're brave, you can tackle a "mango" for a unique taste sensation. Fruit salsa can be made with any chopped fruit or combination of fruits.

Marinara Sauce:

This sauce is a basic Italian ingredient in many recipes and can be dressed up with ground meat, cheese, wine, mushrooms or anything you want. It serves you well in that it has little fat, no fillers, and has a great fresh taste.

> ↪ In a large skillet, put 1 tablespoon **olive oil**

> ↪ When hot, add 1 each thawed bag of chopped **onion** and chopped **green pepper**

> ↪ 2 tablespoons chopped **garlic**

→ **Stir/Cook** for 4 minutes until translucent

→ Add 1 large can chopped or crushed **tomatoes;** bring to a simmer

→ Season with 1 teaspoon each: dried **oregano** and dried **basil**

→ **Salt and pepper to taste**

→ Simmer on low heat, **covered**, for 30 minutes, stirring occasionally. If it's not thick enough, let the sauce simmer uncovered for a few minutes until the desired thickness is reached. Makes approximately 5 cups of sauce, and freezes well.

Pico de Gallo:

This healthy fat-free, fresh sauce is great on eggs, meats, all Mexican dishes, tacos, and burritos and is similar to the salsa you can buy in the store, but its flavor is different and it can be enjoyed on many other foods. It keeps well in a covered container in the refrigerator for about a week. You can add vegetables to make a tasty salad as well.

10 Roma **tomatoes**, chopped

1 Vidalia or sweet **onion**, chopped

½ cup chopped **cilantro**

1 – 2 tablespoons chopped or minced **jalapeno peppers**, picked or fresh (remove the seeds) or use your favorite hot sauce to taste.

Zest of 1 **lime** and the juice of 2 **limes**

Salt/ pepper to taste

Selected References

Andreas, S. (2002) *Transforming Your Self: Becoming Who You Want to Be,* Moab, UT: Real People Press.

Andreas, C. and Andreas, S. (1989) *Heart of the Mind,* Moab, UT: Real People Press.

Bandler, R, (1985) *Using Your Brain for a Change,* Moab, UT: Real People Press.

Bandler, R. and Grinder, J., (1982) *Reframing: Neuro-Linguistic Programming and the Transformation of Meaning,* Moab, UT: Real People Press.

BarnesCare Connection, "Controlling Obesity in the Workplace" http://www.barnescare.com/bcc07, November, 2007

Bennett, B. and Van Vynckt, V. (997) *Dictionary of Healthful Food Terms* Hauppage, NY: Barrons Educational Series.

Bodenhamer, B. G., and L. M. Hall. (1997) *Figuring Out People: Design Engineering with Meta-programs,* Bancyfelin, Wales: Crown House.

Braun Consulting News (2004) "Obesity in the Workplace" http://www.braunconsulting.com/bcg/newsletters/summer2004/summer20043.html

Carroll, L. (1946) *Alice's Adventures in Wonderland and Through the Looking Glass* New York: Macmillan Co..

Centers for Disease Control and Prevention. (2006) "BMI – Body Mass Index: About BMI for Adults", (Available online at www.cdc.gov/ncdcphp/dnpa/bmi/adult_BMI/about_adult_BMI.htm)

Charvet, S. R., (1995) *Words that Change Minds: Mastering the Language of Influence.* Dubuque, IA: Kendall Hunt,

Citrenbaum, C.E., King, M.E., and Cohen, W.I. (*1985*) *Modern Clinical Hypnosis for Habit Control*, New York: W.W. Norton,.

Cochrane G., and Friesen, J., (*1992*) "Hypnotherapy in Weight Loss Treatment". *Journal of Consulting and Clinical Psychology*, 54: 489-92.

Dilts, R. (1990) *Changing Belief Systems with NLP*, Cupertino, CA: Meta Publications,

Dilts, R. (1999) *Sleight of Mouth: The Magic of Conversational Belief Change* Capitola, CA: Meta Publications,

Dilts, R. and J. DeLozier. (2000) *Encyclopedia of Systemic NLP and NLP New Coding.* Scotts Valley, CA: NLP University Press.

Dilts, R., Hallbom T,, and. Smith, S., (1990) *Beliefs: Pathways to Health and Well-Being*, Portland, OR: Metamorphous Press,

Fraser, L., (1997) "The Diet Trap". *Family Therapy Networker,* May-June

Freudenrich, C. C., Ph.D. (2007) *"How Fat Cells Work".* http://health.howstuffworks.com/fat-cell.htm,

Hall, L. M. (2001) *Games Slim People Play.* Grand Junction, CO: Neuro-Semantics,

Harris, C. (1999) *Think Yourself Thin: A Unique Approach to Weight Loss.* Shaftsbury, Dorset, and Boston, MA: Element

Hertz, R., PhD and McDonald, M., PhD (2007) "Obesity in the United States Workforce: Findings from the National Health and Nutrition Examination Surveys (NHANES) III and 1999-2000" *Pfizer Community Health Advocacy.* http://www.communityhealthadvocacy.pfizer.com/programs/**obesity**.asp

Hunt, M. (1984) "Self Hypnosis Works" *Readers Digest,* , April, 164-68,

James, T. and Woodsmall, W. (1988) *Time Line Therapy and the Basis of Personality* Cupertino, CA: Meta Publications.

Knight, S. (2002) *NLP at Work Neuro Linguistic Programming: The Difference that Makes a Difference in Business.* 2nd Edition, Yarmouth, Maine: Brealey Publishing

Knowledge@Wharton (2008) "How Employers Wage War on Workplace Obesity", Forbes.com, (http://www.forbes.com/2008/01/11/obesity-workplace-cdc-ent-hr-cx)

Langer, E. (1997) The Power of Mindful Learning, Cambridge, MA: Da Capo Books,

Lankton, S. and Lankton, C. (1983) *The Answer Within: A Clinical Framework of Ericksonian Hypnotherapy.* New York: Brunner Mazel

McDermott, I and O'Connor, J. (1996) *NLP and Health,* London: Thorsons Publications,

McGraw, P. PhD. (2004) *The Ultimate Weight Solution Food Guide,* NY: Pocket Books

McKenzie, A., PhD, and Walsh, B., MSW. (2004) *The Missing Link to Successful and Permanent Weight Loss* Tigard, OR: Peaceful Pilgrims Press,

Natow, A. PhD, RD and Heslen, J. MA, RD (1995) *The Food Shopping Counter* NY: Pocket Books

Peale, N.V., (1996 reissue) *The Power of Positive Thinking,* New York, NY: Ballentine Books

Racette, S., et al. (2008) "Influence of Weekend Lifestyle Patterns on Body Weight" *Obesity Journal,* 16, 8, 1826–1830.

Rinke, W, (1992) *Make It a Winning Life; Success Strategies for Life, Love, and Business,* Rockville, MD: Achievement Publishers

Roth, G. (1998) *Feeding the Hungry Heart: The Experience of Emotional Eating.* NY: Plume Books

Roth, G. (1989) *Why Weight? A Guide to Ending Compulsive Eating,* NY: Plume Books.

Schwartz, R. (1990) *Diets Still Don't Work,* Galveston, TX. Breakthru Publishing.

Somer, E. MA., RD (1999) *Food and Mood: The Complete Guide to Eating Well and Feeling Your Best* (2nd Edition) NY: Owl Books

Tobey, L. PhD (2001) *The Integrity Moment: Making Powerful Choices in Life* Dubuque, IA: Kendall Hunt Publishing

Van Dusen, A. (2008) "Is Your Weight Holding Back Your Career?" *Forbes.com* (http://www.forbes.com/2008/05/21/health-weight-career-forbeslife-cx)

Wansink, B., Payne, C.R., and Chandon, P. (2007) "Internal and External Cues of Meal Cessation: The French Paradox Redux?" *Obesity,* 15, 12, 2921-2924

Wansink, B. and Payne, C.R., (2008) "Eating Behavior and Obesity at Chinese Buffets" *Obesity, 16* 8, 1957–1960

Wansink, B. (2006) *Mindless Eating: Why We Eat More Than We Think,* New York, NY: Bantam Dell

About the Authors

Jill B. Cody, MA. LCPC

Jill B. Cody, M.A. is a Licensed Clinical Professional Counselor and a Certified Clinical Hypnotherapist. She earned her Masters degree in Counseling Psychology, and has maintained an active private practice in Frederick Maryland since 1978, specializing in goal-oriented counseling and clinical hypnosis. She received her post-graduate training in Clinical Hypnosis and Neuro-Linguistic Programming from the American Hypnosis Training Academy in Silver Spring where she has been a Certified Trainer since 1996. For several years, Jill worked as the Stress Management Instructor for the Wellness Center at Frederick Memorial Hospital. She is the co-author, with Mark Hirschfeld, of ***Collaborative Healing: A "Shorter" Therapy Approach for Survivors of Sexual Abuse.***

A professional member of the National Speakers Association for over ten years, Jill is a dynamic speaker who is noted for her informative and inspiring workshops, seminars and keynote presentations on Winning the Weight War, Effective Interpersonal Communication Skills, and Handling Complaints and Criticism. Jill and her husband, Richard, are the proud parents of three adult sons, and live in Frederick Maryland. She can be reached at www.jillcody.com or by phone at 800-287-5866.

Kip Jawish, NASM, CPT, PAS

Kip has spent a lifetime pursuing excellence in the health and fitness arena. A three-time All State and All-Met football player, in his senior year, Kip was voted All-American at Georgetown Preparatory High School. He was a linebacker on the University of Maryland "Terrapin" football team. After graduation, Kip focused on his personal fitness, and embarked on a career of helping others achieve their fitness goals. He is a veteran of over twenty marathons and a comparable number of triathlons; including the eighty-mile Canadian Death Run with over seventeen thousand feet of elevation changes in the Canadian Rockies. All of this experience gives Kip a unique perspective and diversity in training his clients. He is certified as a personal trainer by the National Academy of Sports Medicine and the American Aerobics International Association, as well as the International Sports Medicine Association. Additionally, Kip is certified by the Egoscue Method as a postural alignment specialist.

In 1989, Kip opened his own Personal Fitness Training studio called "In-Fit Studio". He continues to give speeches and lectures on health and fitness. He can be reached at In-Fit Personal Fitness Studio, www.infitstudio.com or 301-694-0275.

Jane Gross Mercado, M.A., L.C.P.C.

Jane earned her Masters Degree in Counseling Psychology from Hood College in Frederick, Maryland, and has been in private practice for over thirty years. She served as a behaviorist at Frederick Memorial Hospital for their weight management program for four years, during which time she worked intensively helping people who were suffering in their battle with their weight. Many clients in her private practice complained about their weight or body image as their primary concern. Excess weight also contributed to the anxiety, frustration, depression and their lack of confidence, which brought them into counseling in the first place.

She describes herself as *"a 'weight warrior' who had lost many skirmishes with weight, but who is now 'winning that war.' "I am SLOWLY reducing my weight without gaining it back. Historically and genetically, I knew that about two-thirds of my relatives were short and stocky. Clearly,* *this worked against all my efforts to reduce my own weight. After trying most diet programs with continual success, the weight slowly crept back on with a mind-numbing blandness over and over, and **over** again, I have finally found what works to reduce weight successfully over time. The only answer is to change how we think about weight, and then change how we do things every day to initiate and maintain permanent lifestyle changes. I have recorded these insights, discoveries, and actual cooking strategies to help you win your battles."*

Jane can be reached at jmercado7502@yahoo.com.

What Do You Think About This Book?

Please take this opportunity to let me know what you think about this book. Your experience and knowledge are important feedback for me. You can even become an expert contributor. Please take a few minutes to answer the following questions in enough detail, that I have a clear idea of what, why, when, where and how something did (or did not) work for you. If I incorporate your input in the next edition or in another book, I will send you a personalized copy of the book absolutely free. *This questionnaire is also available electronically on my website at* www.wintheweightwar.com.

Jill, the strategies you described in Chapter _____ on pages _____ worked for me.

This is how I used them:

These are the results I got:

Jill, the strategies you described in Chapter ____ on pages _____ did not work for me.

This is how I tried to use them:

These are the results I got:

This is how I fixed it.

Jill, I want to share with you the following personal experiences related to my adventures in Winning the Weight War. Please feel free to use them as you wish.

Your Signature: _____

Date: _____

Your name, complete mailing address and telephone number:

Mail to: Jill Cody
186 Thomas Johnson Dr. #200
Frederick MD 21702

Thank you in advance for taking the time to provide me with your important feedback and/or invaluable experiences.

You and your group will be entertained, inspired, and energized to make transforming changes!

Jill B. Cody, M.A., Licensed Clinical Professional Counselor designs specific stimulating and inspiring keynote presentations, interactive half-day seminars, or informative full-day workshops to help **you**:

WIN THE WEIGHT WAR:

- No-Guilt Restaurant Enjoyment
- Winning Over Temptations
- Conquer Emotional Hunger
- "Fistfull-filling"
- Create a Compelling Future
- Exercise Your Right to be Slender
- Get Rid of the "Losing" Mentality
- Identify Personal Resources and Values of Your Healthy Goal Weight
- "Lunch Box" Psychology

COMMUNICATION SKILLS

- Communicate with Influence
- Build Positive Self-Esteem
- Handle Complaints and Criticism – "Turning Lemons into Lemonade"
- Put MAGIC into Your Relationship

SIX STRESS-LESS STRATEGIES THAT REALLY WORK!

- Assertive Skills for the 21st Century
- Defeating Worry Warts
- Challenging Negative Self Talk
- Understanding and Controlling Pressures
- Self-Hypnosis Strategies to Reduce Stress
- Creating Personal Excellence

Let improved personal or corporate communication skills increase your financial bottom line. Increase your company morale by reducing on- the- job stress. Being in control of your weight increases self-respect, respect of co-workers, and reduces health risks for companies. To schedule a presentation contact Jill Cody at www. jillcody.com or at 800-287-5866

"I guarantee your satisfaction, or there is no fee." - Jill Cody

You will succeed when you put Jill Cody's strategies to work to Win the Weight War!

Order Now!!!

o YES, I want to Win the War on My Weight!

No.	Description	Qty	Price	Total
B101	Win the Weight War: Ten Transforming Perspectives to Take it Off and Keep it Off (Book)		$22.95	
M101	Win the Weight War Flash-Cards (Deck)		$10.95	
A101	Hypnosis Audio CD		$14.95	
V101	Win the Weight War Workshop Video		$49.95	
S102	SUPER BARGAIN: B101 Book, M101 Flashcard Deck, A101 Audio CD, V101 Video: Save 20% on all four.		$79.95	
S103	SUPER BARGAIN: B101 (Book), M101 (Flashcard Deck) Save 15%		$20.95	
S104	SUPER BARGAIN: M101 (Flashcard Deck), A101 - Hypnosis CD. Save 10%		$22.95	
S105	SUPER BARGAIN: B101 (Book), V101 (Video) Save 15%		$62.95	
S106	SUPER BARGAIN: A101 (CD), V101 (Video) Save 15%		$55.95	
	Subtotal			
	If your order is more than $200.00 deduct an additional 10%			
	Maryland residents, add 5% sales tax			
	Shipping and handling $4.50 for the first $50.00; $2.50 f or each additional $50.00 or fraction thereof (outside USA x 2)			
	International orders: Payable in U.S. Funds by MasterCard or Visa credit card Foreign checks – add $10.00 **TOTAL**			

(Overnight shipping available. Call for rates) **Need more than 6 of anything? Call for generous bulk discounts!**

For Faster Service, FAX your credit card charge order to (301) 662-4448 or call (800) 287-5866

YOUR SATISFACTION WITH ALL PRODUCTS IS GUARANTEED!

Please UPS my order to:

Name: _____

Telephone # _____

Company: _____

Address: _____

_____

Payment:

➡ Check or Money Order for the TOTAL amount payable to **Jill B. Cody, M.A. to:**

186 Thomas Johnson Drive, #200
Frederick, MD 21702

➡ MC/Visa card: Please charge $_____ to my MC/Visa card

Number: _____

Exp. Date:_____

Signature: _____

(We need your credit card number, expiration date and your signature to ship your charged order)

Printed in the United States
137846LV00004BA/31/P